THE TOUCH REMEDY

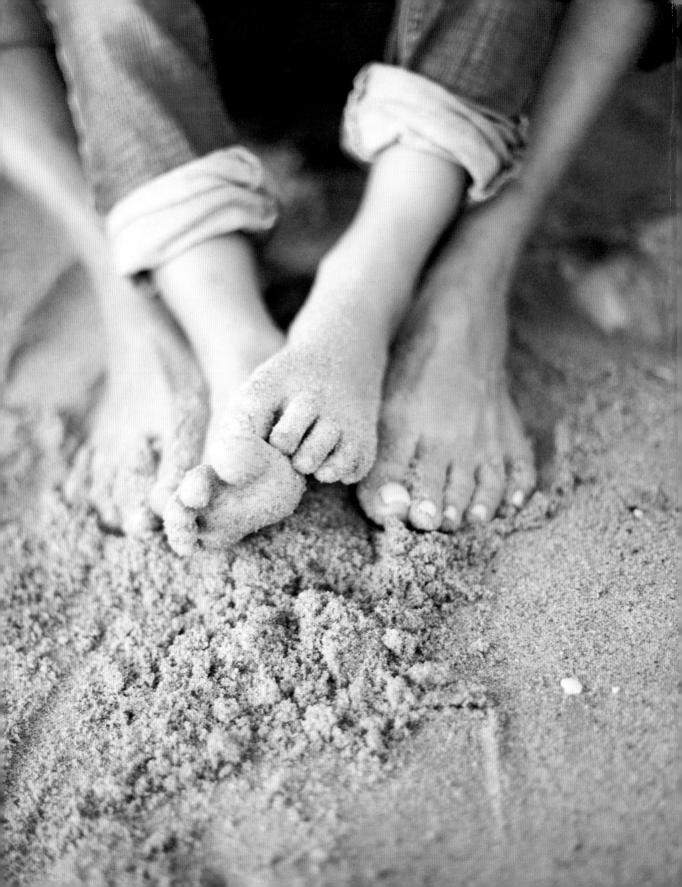

THE TOUCH REMEDY

Hands-On Solutions to De-Stress Your Life

MICHELLE EBBIN

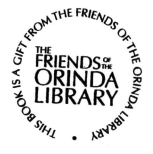

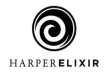

HARPERELIXIR

THE TOUCH REMEDY. Copyright © 2016 by Michelle Ebbin. All rights reserved. No part of this book may be used or reproduced in any manner whatsoever without written permission except in the case of brief quotations embodied in critical articles and reviews. For information address HarperCollins Publishers, 195 Broadway, New York, NY 10007.

HarperCollins books may be purchased for educational, business, or sales promotional use. For information please e-mail the Special Markets Department at SPsales@harpercollins.com.

HarperCollins website: http://www.harpercollins.com

FIRST EDITION

Designed by Campana Design
Photographs by Arna Bajraktarevic; used by permission.

Library of Congress Cataloging-in-Publication Data is available upon request.

ISBN 978–0–06–239245–9

Printed in China

16 17 18 19 20   SCP   10 9 8 7 6 5 4 3 2 1

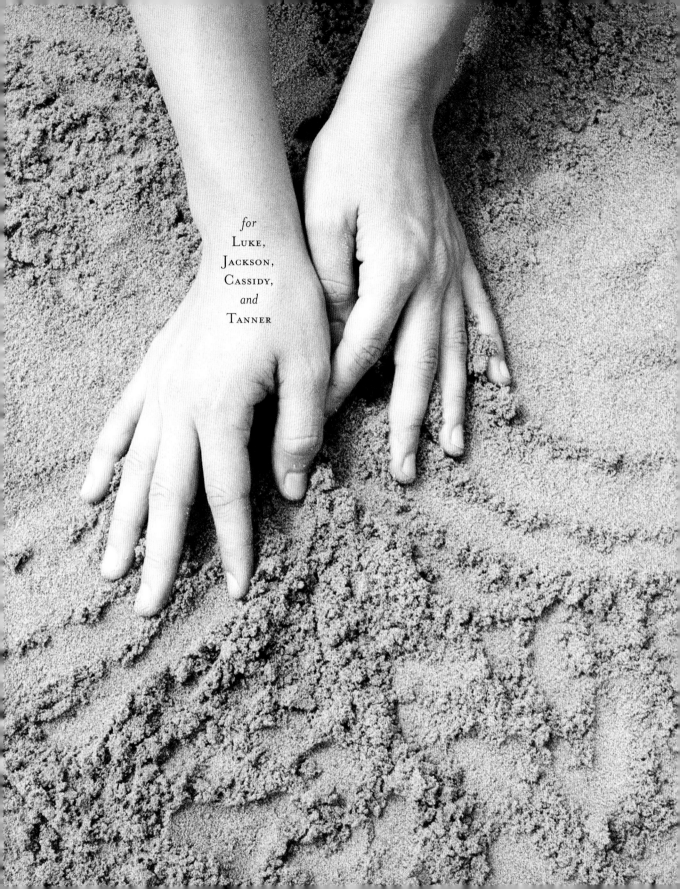

for
LUKE,
JACKSON,
CASSIDY,
and
TANNER

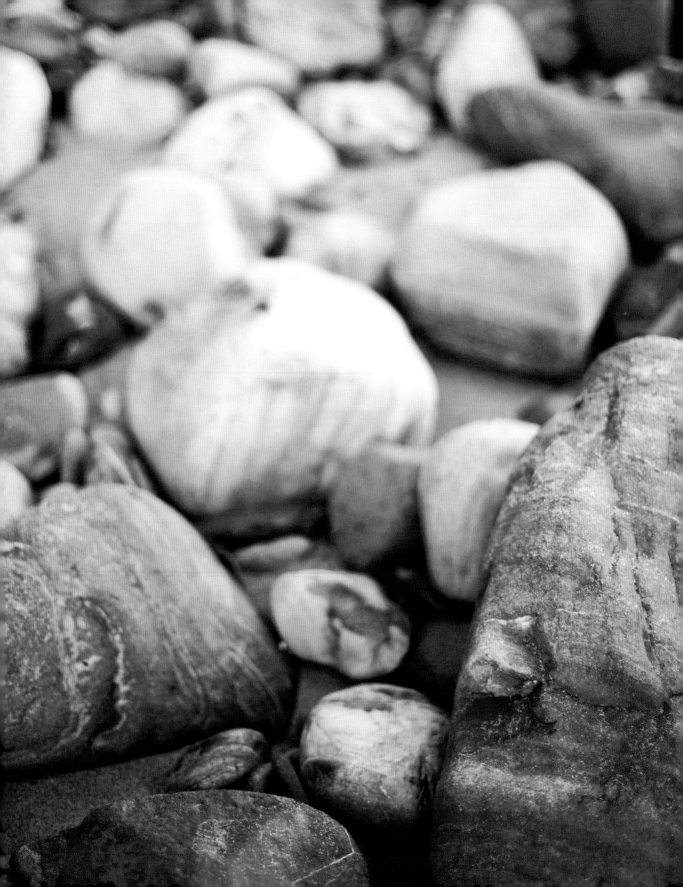

CONTENTS

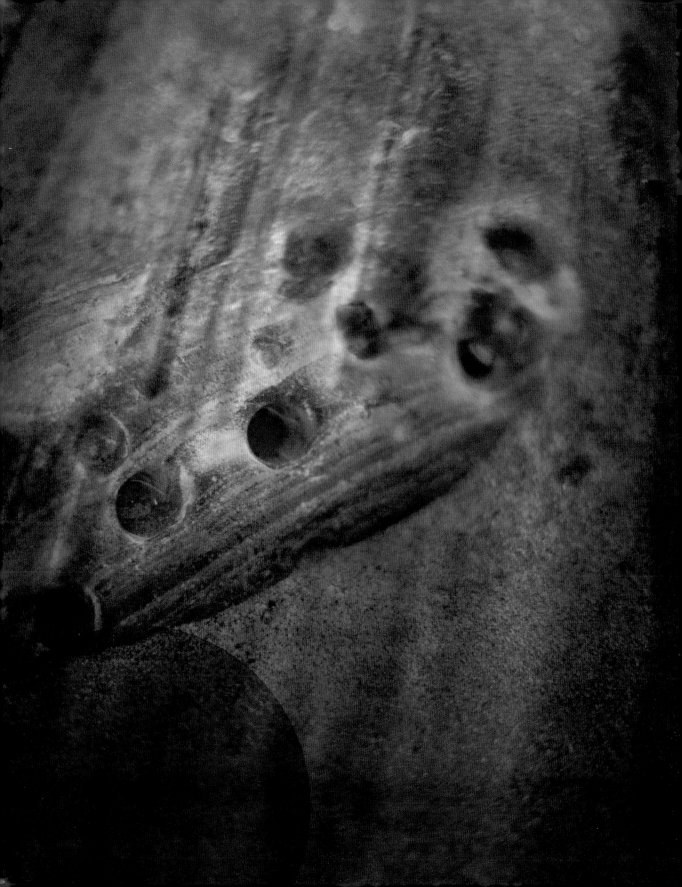

The Touch Remedy

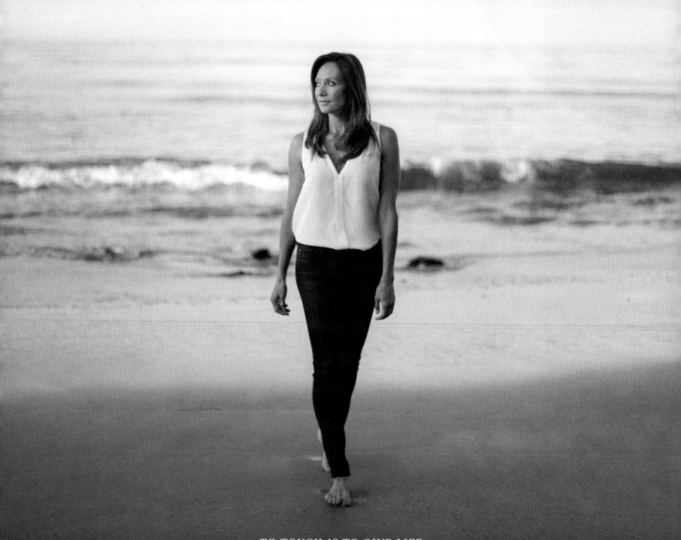

TO TOUCH IS TO GIVE LIFE.

—MICHELANGELO

INTRODUCTION

Welcome to *The Touch Remedy,* a hands-on guide of scientifically proven and personally tested touch-therapy solutions that will help you and your family decrease stress, feel better, and live happier, healthier lives. As a professional massage therapist and, more recently, mother to three young boys, I've continually turned to touch therapies to help myself, my clients, and my family cope with stressful physical and emotional issues. I know how powerful touch can be, and I'm passionate about sharing my knowledge and experience, so that everyone can learn to use touch as an antidote to stress. My message is simple: *touch* can transform lives for the better. With my remedies, you literally can *touch* stress away!

This book is the result of my twenty years practicing and honing the most effective, easy, and safe touch remedies that have worked for me, my family, and the thousands of people I've had the opportunity to touch and teach. There are remedies for everyone, young and old, even pets, and most can be done anywhere, anytime, with nothing but your own two hands. In addition to relieving the negative effects of stress and other common problems, touch remedies improve the intimacy in relationships, deepen family bonds, and communicate love and compassion through touch. By using these remedies regularly on yourself and others you will gain a sense of control over your own and your family's well-being. These are my go-to remedies from my own stress-relief toolbox, and I'm excited to share them with you.

In today's fast-paced world, stress is inevitable, and everyone encounters some form of it on a daily basis. Although a little stress can be beneficial, chronic stress can become emotionally and physically damaging. Stress is related to 99 percent of all illnesses, so it's crucial that we try to do everything in our power to reduce it.[1] Today 26 percent of Americans say they're living with a high level of stress, and 50 percent of American adults say they've suffered a major stressful event in the past year—that's more than 115 million stressed-out people![2]

Stress is contagious, so even if just one member of the family is stressed, the entire family feels the effects. The symptoms of stress—anxiety, irritability,

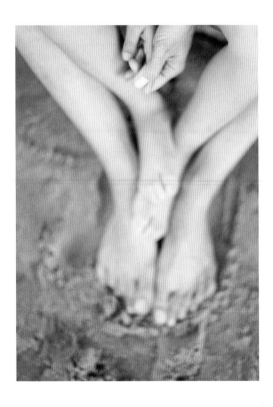

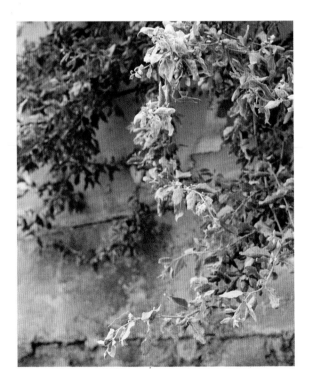

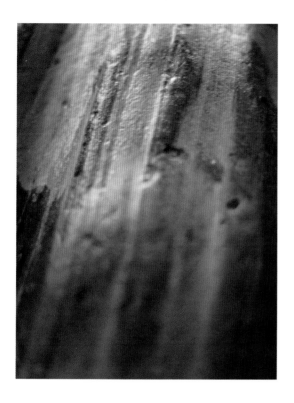

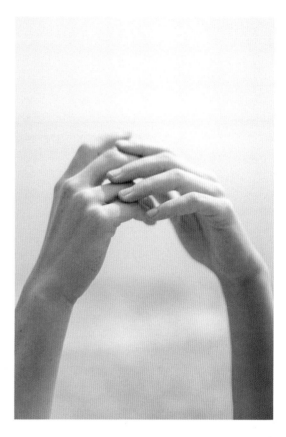

and depression, to name just a few—are almost impossible to hide, and family members are the first to sense when you're under pressure. They not only sense your stress; they inadvertently absorb some of it too. Whether you're an overwhelmed parent or an overworked professional (or both), if you have an irritable baby, a spirited toddler, a hormone-crazed teenager, an exhausted college student, an aging senior, or an anxious pet, you and your family *need* stress relief—and *touch* is the answer.

As a practitioner, I've known that using touch therapy can relax your body, soothe your mind, and improve your relationships, and now there's scientific evidence to prove it. Today research from all over the world confirms the remarkable physical and emotional benefits of touch. Traditional techniques that have been used for centuries finally have clinical data to support them. Studies prove that touch-therapy techniques such as massage, acupressure, and reflexology can relax the nervous system; lower heart rate and blood pressure; ease stress, anxiety, and pain; increase alertness; enhance the immune system; and lessen symptoms of depression. Other studies prove that touch therapy can improve conditions like arthritis, fibromyalgia, and heart disease, ease many cancer-related symptoms, benefit children with ADHD, and improve the quality of life for aging adults.[3]

Massage is increasingly recognized as an alternative medical treatment, and more medical centers nationwide offer massage as a form of patient treatment. In a recent American Hospital Association survey of 1,007 hospitals concerning their use of complementary and alternative medicine therapies, more than 80 percent said they offered massage therapy and over 70 percent said they used massage for pain management and relief.[4] In hospital settings, where the majority of touch is painful and intrusive, massage is an opportunity for patients to experience gentle, soothing touch. New research confirms the importance of human touch as a balance to the high technology of today's health-care practices.[5] I've seen firsthand how touch therapy benefits hospital patients as well as their family members and caregivers, both physically and emotionally. I'm honored to be working with City of Hope, one of the world's leading comprehensive cancer centers, to develop a program that complements mainstream medical care by incorporating touch therapy into the healing process. A portion of the proceeds of this book will go directly to this program.

Touch itself is not only a valuable stress-relieving tool for people of all ages; it's an element vital to our physical and emotional health. In fact, touch is crucial to our early development and all our social interactions. Why? Because touch is not only about physical sensation; it's a means of communicating our emotions nonverbally to one another. According to neuroscientists, we have an innate ability to decode emotions via touch. Even the simplest of touches, say a hand on your arm or a pat on your back, has a powerful effect on your brain.[6] Momentary touches can communicate an even wider range of emotion than hand gestures or facial expressions and sometimes do so more quickly and accurately than words. So if inadvertent touch can affect you, just imagine the powerful effect that intentional, compassionate touch therapy can have!

The bad news is that scientists also report that American society is dangerously touch-deprived, and most Americans today are in desperate need of a one-on-one connection.[7] Studies show that most people in the United States have limited daily one-on-one contact with anyone other than their spouse or partner, and we touch each other less than people in many other cultures. This lack of touch, also known as "skin hunger," creates not only more stress, but a host of other problems, including anxiety, mood disorders, depression, and a weakened immune system. People who don't get enough touch are lonelier and less happy, have less social support and lower relationship satisfaction, and are more likely to have an impaired ability to express and interpret emotion, a condition called alexithymia. This makes them less likely to form secure attachments with others in their lives.[8] People who don't get enough touch also miss out on the benefits of oxytocin, the "feel-good" hormone that's released in your body when you touch or are touched, which lowers cortisol levels, reduces stress and pain, and makes people feel secure and trusting toward each other.

Unfortunately, "skin hunger" isn't an extreme condition; rather, it's a very common experience that many people have at different times in their lives. According to the Urban Dictionary, "When you've been without a date for a long, long time, haven't seen your mom for ages, and no one has hugged you forever and you need someone to touch and hug you, that's skin hunger. . . . When you are lying in bed or sitting on a park bench and begin fantasizing about lying in bed holding another person and *not* thinking about sex, that's skin hunger."[9]

My goal in writing this book is to increase awareness about the collective problem of touch deprivation, to awaken you to the tremendous benefits of touch, and to inspire you to improve your health by bringing more touch into your life. I hope to transform our current culture of touch by encouraging you to recognize touch as a necessity rather than a luxury and motivating you to reach out and touch more often using touch remedies. My intention is to inspire a *touch revolution* that brings touch therapy to the forefront of traditional stress management for individuals, families, and company health programs everywhere.

Over the last two decades, scientific evidence has helped the ancient practices of yoga, meditation, and mindfulness gain mainstream acceptance, and they're now practiced by millions of people worldwide. The time has come for touch therapy to take its place beside these effective tools for stress relief and healthy living. Touch is a powerful healer, and the remedies in this book will get you started on your own *touch revolution*.

Touch can improve every part of your life. I know this is true because, besides the research to prove it, I experienced life-changing effects through my own touch revolution. Over the years, whether it was reflexology to cure a headache or hangover, acupressure to help my husband's aching back, or baby massage to ease my infant's colic, touch has played a key role in maintaining my family's optimal health and well-being. However, I was not always so touch-inclined and until my mid-twenties I had no idea that touch therapy could be so useful or effective. Instead, I came upon it out of necessity.

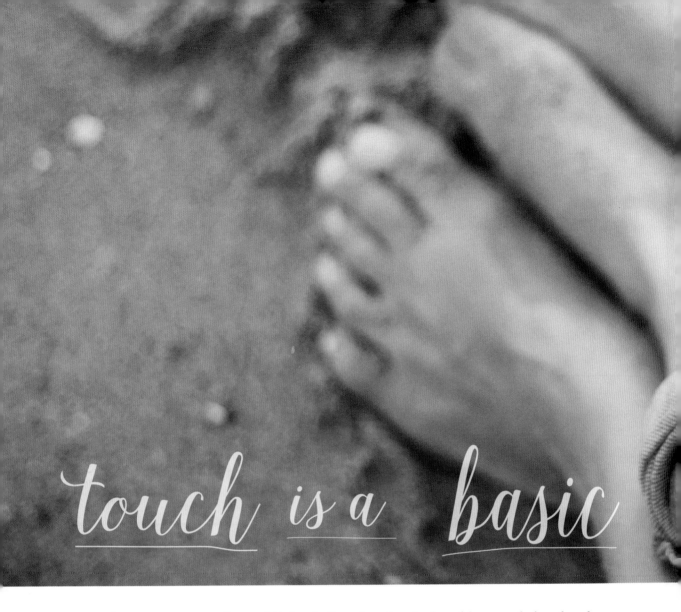

touch is a basic

When I was twenty-five and living in Los Angeles, I often felt overwhelmed and completely stressed out about my future and what I was going to do with the rest of my life. Much to the chagrin of my parents, who had sent me to the prestigious boarding school Phillips Academy Andover and then on to Columbia University with the expectation that I would have a traditional career, I chose a different course. After a brief stint working in the corporate world and quickly realizing it was not for me, I went back to doing what I knew and loved, dance.

Although I had practiced ballet since I was five years old, in the mid-1980s I fell in love with hip-hop. It was MTV's music video heyday and, living in New York, I danced my way through several fun years of hip-hop and rap videos alongside the likes of JLo, Heavy D,

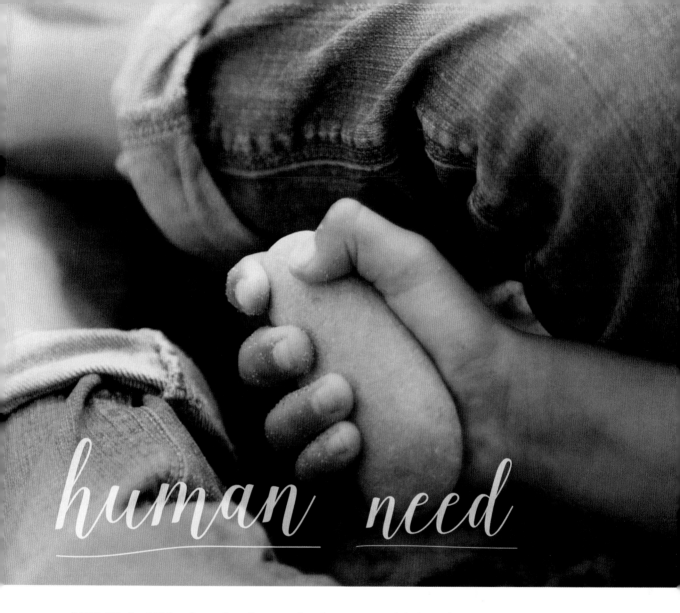

human need

and EPMD. In 1992, after a few dance-related injuries and feeling that I wanted to experience a world outside of NYC, I moved to Los Angeles ready to try something new and figure out the rest of my life. This is when the stress set in.

As a single girl with few responsibilities, I couldn't understand why and how stress could have such a profound effect on me. As many friends turned to alcohol, drugs, and other mind-numbing habits, I realized that in order to avoid the stress roller coaster, I had to look inward to figure out what my stressors were and deal with them in a natural, sustainable way. I immersed myself in one New Age practice after another: yoga, meditation, crystal healing, colonics, ear candling, sweat lodges. . . . You name it, I tried it. As a former dancer, I was drawn to therapies that could connect my body and mind and cultivate a sense of calm. A friend suggested bodywork, and after my very first massage, which relaxed my body and mind to a state of tranquility I'd never felt before, I was hooked. I made it my mission to learn everything I could about touch.

I enrolled at the Institute of Psycho-Structural Balancing in Los Angeles, and from there I began my massage therapy practice, quickly building a following of great clients mainly in the entertainment industry. In 1995 I founded Basic Knead, a business that dispatched massage therapists to Hollywood studios and sets. At the same time, I started thinking of unique ways to teach a broader array of people how to bring touch into their lives frequently and affordably. In 1997 I created my first product, the original Reflexology Sox, which are socks that detail the reflex points to press on the soles of your feet to affect different parts of the body, and within six months sold over twenty thousand pairs (and later over five hundred thousand pairs). My touch-therapy career continued to grow, and in addition to running Basic Knead and marketing my Reflexology Sox, I began creating other massage products, books, and DVDs, all designed to encourage people to touch more and cultivate a healthier lifestyle.

Since then, I've nurtured and witnessed thousands of instances of touch therapy transforming lives, both physically and emotionally. Touch is a basic human need, one that shouldn't be overlooked. Many people may not be able to afford or have the free time for professional massage, but everyone can and should take a few minutes each day to nurture themselves with touch. Just like yoga or meditation, touch therapy *is* something you can practice at home to great effect—it is an affordable, accessible, DIY self-care tool you can use daily, and this book will teach you how. The earlier we learn and begin practicing stress-relieving self-care, the more we benefit throughout our lives. It's never too late. In this book, you'll find touch remedies for people at every stage of life.

Many of us take prescription drugs to stabilize our moods and manage stress. And although these drugs are lifesaving for many, I do believe that consistent practice of touch remedies can supplement such regimens and, for some, lessen our reliance on prescription medications. The touch remedies in this book not only bring immediate relief; they can help our bodies tap into the power to heal themselves. Touch techniques like acupressure, reflexology, Thai massage (partner massage), cranial-sacral therapy, deep-tissue massage, lymphatic massage, Swedish massage, trigger-point therapy (self-myofascial release), and therapeutic touch counteract the hazards of living with too much stress and not enough touch. My simple instructions and descriptions will demystify all of these techniques and motivate you to use them as part of your own self-care practice.

Science proves that we all have a fundamental need to touch and be touched. Truth be told, we could all use an extra hug, or better yet a soothing foot massage, every now and then. With *The Touch Remedy* I aim to promote awareness of the important role that simple, daily touch plays in leading happy, healthy lives—and to empower you to take your well-being quite literally into your own hands with conscious, intentional, compassionate touch. The *touch revolution* I envision is about recognizing the scientific evidence for the significance of touch and sparking a new approach to mainstream health-care practices that incorporates one proven antidote to stress, *touch*.

With the touch remedies in this book, you really can transform your life. Just as stress is contagious, touch can be contagious too, making you and everyone around you happier, healthier, and more connected. I invite you to start your own touch revolution with a call to action: *To inspire and cultivate more touch in the world.* So go ahead, harness the power that lies within the palms of your hands and touch someone today. Touch more, stress less.

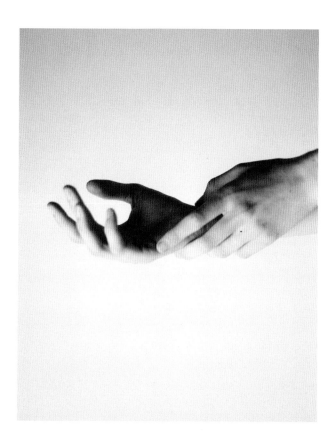

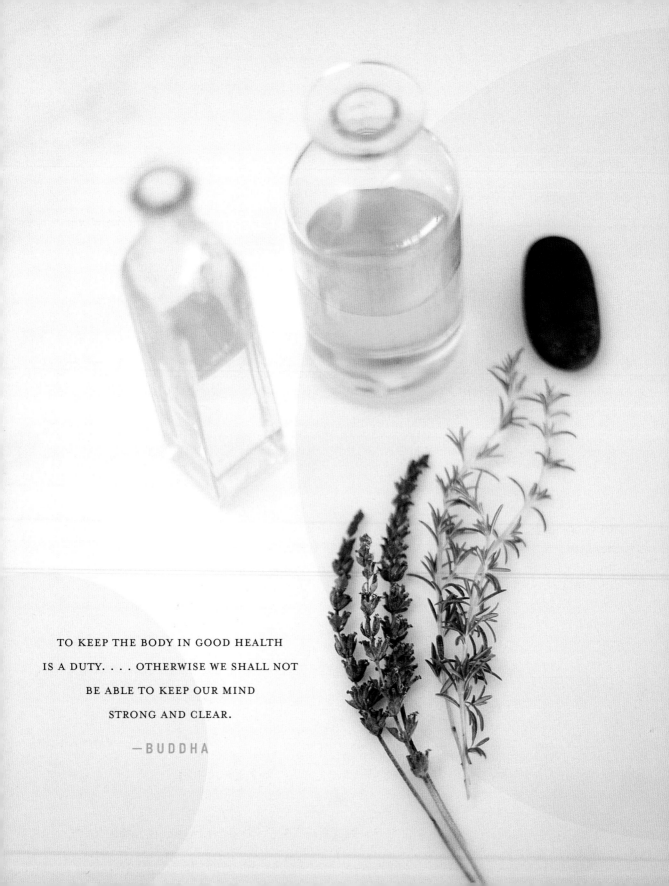

TO KEEP THE BODY IN GOOD HEALTH
IS A DUTY. . . . OTHERWISE WE SHALL NOT
BE ABLE TO KEEP OUR MIND
STRONG AND CLEAR.

—BUDDHA

CHAPTER ONE

Touch-Therapy Techniques and Tools

What is touch therapy? There are hundreds of different types of touch therapies (thirteen in this book alone), and although they differ from each other greatly with regard to pressure and technique, they all share the same holistic philosophy: *The way to achieve optimal health is by gaining proper balance in life*. Like other complementary medicines, all touch therapies are "holistic" in that they consider the whole person—body, mind, spirit, and emotions—in the quest for optimal health and wellness.

Before I explain each technique, I'd like to clearly define what I mean by "touch therapy." Traditionally, when people talk about touch therapy, they're referring specifically to therapeutic touch or "energy therapy," in which a practitioner's hands are placed on or just above a patient's body to rebalance the body's energy and relieve stress and discomfort. However, in this book, for the purpose of drawing attention to the importance of touch, I will be using "touch therapy" as a catch-all term for *all the systematic healing techniques that involve using touch to relax the body and soothe the mind.* As you read each chapter, the different touch-therapy techniques will be explained in greater detail as they apply to specific remedies.

Touch-Therapy Techniques

Before you begin to use the touch remedies in each chapter, it's helpful to understand what each touch-therapy technique is all about, how the techniques differ from each other, why you'd use one technique and its remedy instead of another for a specific problem—and how healing through touch can happen in your own body. Each technique has its own unique philosophy and history, but they're all based on the holistic idea that every part of your body is intimately interconnected with every other part, so they treat the "whole person," not just the physical symptoms of a problem. While all of the techniques in each of the chapters offer general stress relief, for the most effective results I recommend using the specific remedies designated to resolve particular needs.

touch relaxes the body and soothes the mind

Acupressure

Acupressure is one of my favorite therapies to use and teach, because it's something you can easily do to yourself or someone else anytime, anywhere. It's similar to acupuncture, but instead of needles it uses manual pressure applied (usually with your fingertips) to specific points on your body.

Developed over five thousand years ago as an important part of traditional Chinese medicine, acupressure is based on the concept that our body has life energy, called *chi* or *qi,* which flows through fourteen invisible lines, called meridians, that connect our organs to other parts of our body. Acupuncture and acupressure points lie on these meridians, and by stimulating specific points you can elicit a response from the nervous system that can improve blood flow, enhance the flow of energy, release tension, promote deep relaxation, and unblock any congestion of life energy within the body.

According to Chinese philosophy, illness and disease are caused by an obstruction in the flow of energy along a meridian. By applying pressure to certain points you can unblock the energy and alleviate many acute and chronic problems, including nausea, fatigue, headaches, stomachaches, menstrual cramps, back pain, and muscle tension.

Aromatherapy

I love aromatherapy. I use it every day on myself and my kids (lavender and rose geranium are my go-to scents). This complementary and alternative therapy uses essential oils and other aromatic plant compounds to alter mood and to improve physical and emotional health. It's often used in conjunction with massage to further relax the body and mind.

The theory behind it is that the inhalation of essential oils stimulates the part of the brain connected to smell (the olfactory system), which then sends a signal to the limbic system, which controls emotions and retrieves memories. This causes the body to release chemicals that can make you feel many different ways: relaxed, calm, energized, sensual, or simply happy, just to name a few. Aromatherapy essential oils are said to have a direct pharmacological effect.

I recommend going on a scent journey at your local health store and inhaling many different essential oils. Use the ones that you're drawn to first. For use on the skin, always add a few drops of essential oil to a few ounces of an unscented, natural vegetable oil (called a "carrier" oil), such as almond or grapeseed oil. Do *not* put essential oil directly onto your skin, as essential oils are very potent and may cause burning or stinging.

Baby Massage

As a certified infant massage instructor and mother of three, I truly believe that every parent and every person who cares for a baby needs to learn baby massage. This therapy helps parents and caregivers soothe, nurture, and bond with a new baby. Baby massage is an ancient parenting tradition in many cultures, one that's gaining popularity in our culture today. Many hospitals are now including it in their neonatal programs.

The technique of baby massage is a gentle, rhythmic stroking of your baby's body and head (oil or lotion is optional) along with gentle stretching of the arms and legs. It's a relaxing form of nonverbal communication that helps you express love and care for your baby and enhances parent-child attachment. Research has demonstrated that nurturing touch for infants is critical in establishing the foundation of their psychological well-being.

The amazing benefits of baby massage include increased weight gain, better digestion (which means less crying), improved circulation, teething pain relief, and better sleep. The benefits for parents can last a lifetime. Beyond enhancing intimacy and promoting attachment, baby massage can increase parents' confidence and improve communication with their baby.

I used baby-massage techniques on my three boys from the day they were born, and it helped tremendously then, as massage still does today. I had reliable techniques that I could use to help soothe their tummies when they had gas and comfort them when they were irritable and restless. Today, my boys still ask for back and foot massages to help them relax and go to sleep. The best thing is that they are all comfortable in their bodies, and they love to touch and be touched.

Cranial-Sacral Therapy

This is my go-to therapy when I have a headache that lasts for more than a day. Cranial-sacral therapy (CST) is an extremely gentle, noninvasive healing technique that's based on applying very light pressure (no more than the weight of a nickel) to the head, neck, and spine. By decompressing these areas, CST can improve the flow of spinal fluid between the head and the sacrum and release tension in the soft tissues that surround the central nervous system. This nourishes the brain and soothes the nervous system, so you can deeply relax and your body can heal itself.

CST can relieve pain, release tension, improve your overall well-being, and help you stay balanced so that your body functions better. It can be used for many chronic and acute problems, including migraines and headaches, neck and back pain, fibromyalgia, stress- and tension-related disorders, central nervous system disorders, temporomandibular joint dysfunction (TMJD), scoliosis, autism, ADD/ADHD, posttraumatic stress disorder (PTSD), and more.

Deep-Tissue Massage

Deep-tissue massage is my preferred touch-therapy technique when I'm working out regularly. It's not for everyone, since it can be a bit painful, but it's very effective in releasing chronic muscle tension and increasing circulation to areas that may be tight or tender. In addition to hands, you can use elbows, forearms, and even your feet to apply pressure. Similar to Swedish massage, deep-tissue massage uses some of the same strokes, but the movements are slower and the pressure is deeper and more focused to reach the sublayer of muscles, tendons, and fascia (the connective tissue surrounding muscles, bones, and joints).

When you have chronic muscle tension or an injury, adhesions (bands of painful, rigid tissue) often develop in your muscles that can slow circulation, limit movement, and cause pain and inflammation. Deep-tissue massage breaks down these adhesions to relieve pain and restore normal circulation and movement. It's especially helpful for chronic pain and muscle tension (in back, legs, neck, shoulders), recovery from injuries (including repetitive strain injuries such as carpal tunnel syndrome), sciatica, fibromyalgia, and more. A recent study found that deep-tissue massage has a positive effect on reducing pain in patients with chronic lower-back pain.[1]

Lymphatic Massage

Lymphatic massage is a technique I use when I'm feeling sluggish and heavy and want to energize my body (which is every day!). Also known as manual lymphatic drainage (MLD) or lymph-drainage therapy (LDT), lymphatic massage is a very gentle technique that stimulates your body's lymphatic system and results in deep relaxation, detoxification, and healing.

The lymphatic system, a part of the circulatory system, is a network of tissues and organs that runs throughout your body. It's composed of tiny tubes called lymphatic vessels, lymph nodes, and lymph fluid as well as the tonsils, adenoids, spleen, and thymus. This powerful system drains the clear lymph fluid from tissues and moves it in the direction of the heart to the subclavian veins near the collarbones, where it reenters the bloodstream. As lymph fluid moves through the body, bacteria and other microbes are picked up and trapped inside lymph nodes, where they can be attacked and destroyed by white blood cells. Before being emptied into the blood, lymph fluid is filtered through the spleen, thymus, and lymph nodes.

The lymphatic system has several functions. It manages fluid levels in the body by returning excess fluid from tissues to the blood. It absorbs and transports fats and fatty acids from the digestive system. It transports white blood cells to and from the lymph nodes. Finally, it helps rid the body of toxins, bacteria, waste, and other unwanted materials to help your immune system defend against invading viruses and disease.

Occasionally, conditions such as illness, stress, poor diet, and surgery can overload the lymphatic system, so that it becomes lethargic and inefficient. By manually stimulating the lymphatic system through light pressure and rhythmic circular movements with your hands or a dry soft-bristled brush (which is where the term "dry brushing" comes from), you can accelerate the lymph system, allowing it to process up to ten times more fluid than normal. This enhances the "lymphatic flow" that filters out waste products, dead cells, excess proteins, and toxins from the tissues, increases the production of lymphocytes, which increases your body's ability to fight infections, and activates the parasympathetic response, producing a body-wide relaxation effect. In addition, it can help reduce bloating, improve your skin, fight cellulite, and help you look and feel better.

A recent study shows that MLD is effective in reducing the activity of the sympathetic nervous system (SNS).[2] The SNS is responsible for the body's fight-or-flight response to stress, which includes increased heart rate and respiration, increased perspiration and blood pressure, and slowed digestion. Reducing SNS activity can help lessen these negative effects in the body, which is particularly helpful when stress is ongoing. (You should avoid lymphatic massage if you have lymphedema and notice an increase in swelling, lymphangitis, congestive heart failure, or pain.)

Oncology Massage

Oncology massage consists of modified massage-therapy techniques that take into account the complications of cancer and cancer treatment. Massage therapists who are trained in oncology massage have an informed understanding of the disease and how it can affect the body, the side effects of cancer treatments, and how to safely modify massage techniques according to the particular form of the disease and what's going on with the individual patient.

Massage during cancer treatment is extremely beneficial, and I believe it should be available to every cancer patient. Although some hospitals currently offer in- and out-patient oncology therapy, it's not as accessible as it should be. Over the past few years I've been working with City of Hope, a leading cancer center in California, to bring oncology massage to more patients. I've led workshops teaching simple and very safe techniques that everyone can do at home to relax patients undergoing cancer treatment. In Chapter 9, I'll explain several touch-therapy techniques that family, friends, and caregivers can safely do to relax cancer patients before, after, and even during treatment.

Pregnancy Massage

Pregnancy massage was a lifesaver for me during my three pregnancies, as it was the only time I felt I could really relax. Also known as prenatal or postnatal massage, pregnancy massage is the common term for any hands-on massage before, during, or after pregnancy. This safe technique is similar to regular Swedish massage, as it relaxes muscles, eases sore areas, and improves circulation and mobility, but it uses positions (such as lying on one's side) and movements that are modified to meet the needs of pregnant women and their changing bodies.

With a growing uterus and shifts in hormonal levels and metabolism, pregnancy is a time of both physical and emotional changes, and almost every pregnant woman experiences some kind of discomfort during pregnancy. The pregnancy-massage partner techniques in this book can help ease many of these problems, including headaches, backaches, nausea, fatigue, moodiness, difficulty sleeping, and swollen ankles and legs. In addition to decreasing stress and promoting relaxation, it's also a great way for partners, family, and friends to emotionally support a mom-to-be at a time when she needs it the most.

Reflexology

Reflexology is so much more than a foot massage! It's an ancient healing technique based on the theory that every single part of your body is connected, through nerve pathways, to your *hands, feet,* and *ears.* By pressing on specific points, called reflexes, on your hands, feet, or ears, you can elicit a response from the nervous system that can improve the flow of energy in your body, relieve stress, reduce pain, increase your energy, boost your immune system, increase blood circulation, promote healing, and improve your overall well-being.

Reflexology essentially clears energy pathways that have been blocked. The reflexology chart on p. 21 can show you where to press to stimulate specific parts of the body that may need help. As you feel your feet, hands, or ears, tender areas or places that feel like grains of sand may indicate a weakness or imbalance in the corresponding part of the body. Pay attention to sensitive areas, as they need stimulation the most. Also, remember to stimulate the same points on *both* feet (if you're working on the feet) and *both* hands (if you're working on the hands), so you aren't left feeling imbalanced. Most of the points are on the same place on both feet, with the exception of the heart, which is only on the left foot, and the liver, which is only on the right foot. As you read through each chapter, refer to the reflexology chart to help you locate specific reflex points.

Reflexology is a great therapy to use on yourself, since you can easily reach your own hands and feet, as well as on people who may be self-conscious about their body. Most important, it feels amazing!

According to a study at the University of Portsmouth, reflexology may be as effective as painkillers. Researchers found that participants in the study felt about 40 percent less pain and were able to withstand pain for 45 percent longer, when they used reflexology as a method for pain relief.[3]

Swedish Massage

Swedish massage is the most common and best-known massage technique, and it can be both relaxing and energizing. I enjoy it when I want a soothing massage rather than a deeper, more painful massage. Swedish massage uses oil or lotion and involves long soft, gliding, and kneading strokes as well as light rhythmic tapping strokes on the topmost layers of muscles, with pressure that varies from light to firm. Often combined with manipulation and stretching of the limbs, it relieves muscles tension, improves circulation, and helps heal injuries. The four most common strokes of Swedish massage are:

> *Effleurage:* a smooth, gliding stroke to relax soft tissue

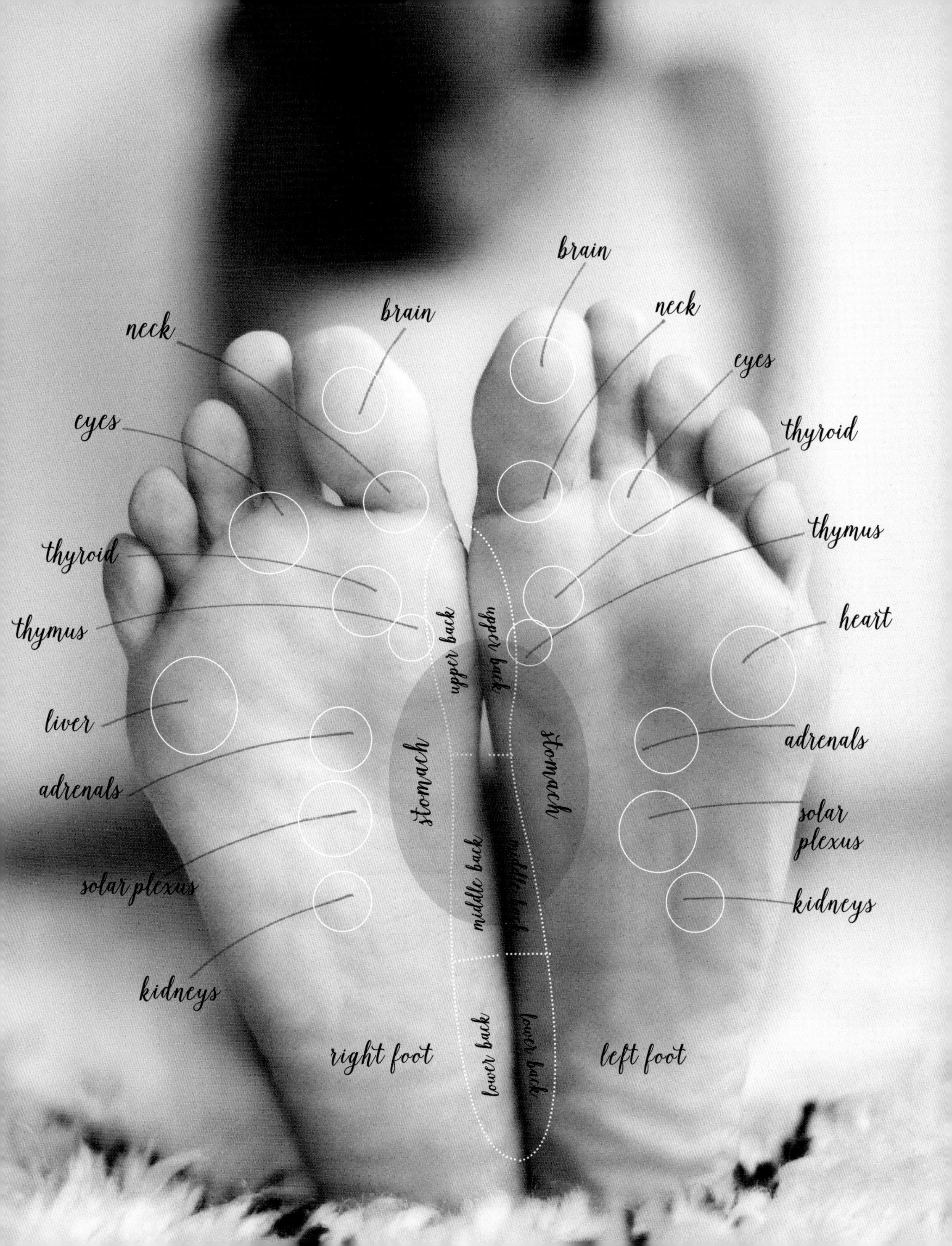

brain

neck

brain

neck

eyes

eyes

thyroid

thyroid

thymus

thymus

heart

liver

upper back

upper back

adrenals

stomach

stomach

adrenals

solar plexus

solar plexus

middle back

middle back

kidneys

kidneys

right foot

lower back

lower back

left foot

Petrissage: rhythmic kneading, squeezing, or rolling of the skin

Friction: more targeted, deep circular movements on specific areas that cause muscle fibers to rub against each other, which increases blood flow and can break down scar tissue

Percussion: short choppy tapping done with cupped hands, fingers, or the edge of the hand to stimulate the body, which is often done at the very end of a massage

Thai Massage, or Partner Massage

Many of the partner-massage techniques I use in this book are variations of Thai massage, a main branch of Thai traditional medicine considered by practitioners to be a medical treatment for a wide variety of ailments, including asthma, migraines, anxiety, physical and emotional stress, muscle tension and tightness, blocked energy, and sleep disorders. In Thailand, Thai massage is actually part of the training program for traditional Thai physicians.

This full-body massage, which focuses on clearing up blockages along the body's energy lines and thus stimulating the flow of blood and lymph throughout the body, is my favorite way to get deep into tight muscles with the least amount of effort. The technique is similar to yoga, as it involves yoga-like positions and stretches, rhythm and joint mobilization, and deep compression using your hands, feet, and elbows. Unlike other touch-therapy techniques in which there is more skin-to-skin contact and the receiver is encouraged to zone out and relax, this technique requires keeping clothes on to allow for manipulation of the body and encourages more engagement and communication between the massage giver and receiver.

Many of the positions and stretches benefit both people. That's why it's also referred to as partner massage. In addition to deep relaxation, increased flexibility, and improved energy, Thai massage can deepen the connection between you and your partner and inspire compassion and trust. I love it because it's a technique that relaxes *you,* the giver of the massage, as much as the receiver!

Therapeutic Touch

Therapeutic Touch (commonly shortened to TT) is an energy therapy that promotes healing and reduces pain and anxiety. It relies on tapping into the energy, or "life force," that surrounds us and is available to us at all times to create balance and wellness. This energy has been known by dozens of names over thousands of years. It is called *chi* in China, *ki* in Japan, *prana* in Hindu and Tibetan cultures, *mana* in Polynesia, and *baraka* in North Africa. The concept of energy therapy is both rational and straightforward. It's based on the theory that diseases and disorders alter the electromagnetic properties of molecules, cells, tissues, and organs, and energy therapy, including therapeutic touch, can help to positively affect any unbalanced parts of the body.[4]

Rather than applying pressure to the skin, this technique is based on placing your hands on or just above a person's body, feeling the energy field (often felt as warmth or heat) in that area, and smoothing out any energy imbalances with gentle, soothing hand motions. Similar to Reiki, TT is a means of transferring healing energy to someone who needs it. It's safe for everyone, especially the elderly and anyone battling an illness, as it subtly rebalances the body's *chi* (energy flow).

TT has many healing benefits, including improving conditions such as pain, fever, swelling, infections, wounds, ulcers, thyroid problems, colic, burns, nausea, PMS, diarrhea, and headaches. It's been used to treat the symptoms of anxiety, Alzheimer's, AIDS, asthma, autism, multiple sclerosis, stroke, comas, and cancer. In a 2003 study, TT lowered pain, blood pressure, fatigue, and emotional problems in cancer patients receiving chemotherapy.[5] Thousands of health-care professionals, mostly nurses, have learned TT worldwide, and it's a technique that everyone can learn to do at home.

Trigger-Point Therapy, or Self-Myofascial Release

Trigger-Point Therapy, or Self-Myofascial Release (SMR), often causes people to say, "Aaahh, it hurts so good." It's based on applying concentrated pressure to specific tight areas within muscle tissue, called "trigger points" (everyone has them), that cause pain and stiffness in other parts of the body. For example, a trigger point in your neck may cause a headache, and a trigger point in your back may cause shoulder pain. Trigger points themselves are adhesions, or "knots," in your muscles that develop from small tears caused by overstressing the muscles, either through overuse or trauma. When muscle tears don't heal properly, the layers of fascia can adhere together in knots, which causes pain and restricts your range of motion.

Through trigger-point therapy you can heal yourself by identifying and activating specific trigger points on your own body that cause pain. Through cycles of isolated pressure and release, you can open tight areas in your muscles and naturally alleviate pain, stiffness, and stress. Personally, trigger-point therapy works like magic on certain areas of my neck and has prevented countless migraines from ruining my day!

Touch-Remedy Tools

Although most of the remedies in this book can be done with nothing but your own two hands, some people find they prefer the soothing "glide" of oil or lotion on their hands as they massage. And there are a few remedies in these pages that require simple tools—household items, for the most part—that you probably already have at home. Don't worry—you really don't need many tools at all to achieve relaxing, healing, stress-relieving results! But, as always, it's good to be prepared, so here's my list.

Massage Oil

I recommend all-natural, organic (food-grade, if possible), unscented vegetable oils such as almond, jojoba, or grapeseed oil. You can always add aromatherapy essential oils to unscented oil. The skin is our body's largest organ, and it absorbs the majority of what we put onto it. My belief is that if you're going to put something *on* your body, you should be able to put it *in* your

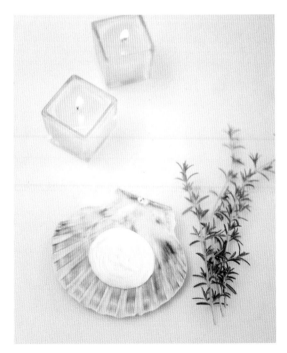

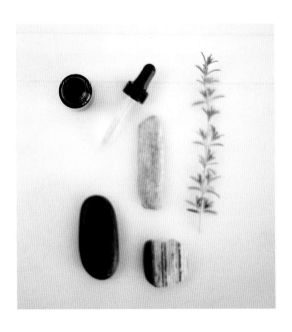

body. Massage oil and lotion will help your hands glide smoothly over the body and, at the same time, will nourish the skin. I prefer to use massage oil because it glides better than lotion. However, for deep-tissue massage, when I want more control and less "slipperiness," I use lotion.

Massage Lotion

I recommend organic, paraben-free lotions. Recently, scientific studies have shown that several chemicals commonly found in personal-care products, including lotions, are potentially harmful to the body, can disrupt the hormone system and cause allergies, and may accelerate cancer. To be on the safe side, read ingredient labels and try to avoid lotions that contain:

> Phthalates
> Propylene glycol
> Mineral oil
> PABA
> Petrolatum
> Paraffin DEA
> Sodium lauryl sulfates
> Synthetic fragrances
> Artificial colors

Aromatherapy Essential Oils

Adding a few drops of aromatherapy oils to unscented oil or lotion can give your massage extra *zing*. I love relaxing and rejuvenating scents like lavender, rosemary, Roman chamomile, and rose geranium. Experiment with your favorite scents. Depending on how strong you want your oil to smell, I suggest adding 2 to 4 drops of essential oil to 2 ounces of unscented, natural "carrier" oil, such as almond, grapeseed, or sesame.

hands are the best tools.

Soft-Bristled Brush

A natural, soft-bristled brush, ideally with a long handle so you can reach every part of your body, is very helpful for dry brushing your skin. Dry brushing is a form of lymphatic massage that stimulates the lymph system and can help the body rid itself of toxins, increase circulation, and improve your energy level. You brush in the direction of the heart with clockwise circular motions, beginning at the feet and moving up your body. I like to do this every morning before jumping in the shower as well as anytime I'm feeling sluggish for a quick rejuvenating pick-me-up.

Tennis Balls (2)

A tennis ball is a great massage tool to use when you want to relieve soreness and pain, and increase circulation in your own body. When you can't get to a massage therapist and there's no one around to rub those hard-to-reach places (such as your back, neck, or hamstrings), rolling on a tennis ball can help you work the deepest layers of muscle and connective tissue to dissolve knots and stretch your muscles. In this book, tennis balls are used in several deep-tissue and cranial-sacral self-remedies.

Foam Roller

A foam roller is my go-to tool for self-myofascial release, a technique you can do to break down knots in your muscles, boost circulation, increase flexibility, and melt away stress. The roller gets to the fascia of your muscles in a similar way as a deep-tissue massage, working out toxins and scar tissue and restructuring the muscles. Rollers are approximately 6 inches in diameter and vary in firmness (the firmer the roller, the deeper the massage.) These are available at most sporting-goods stores and online. I highly recommend everyone stash away a foam roller in the closet—they're essential to deep-tissue self-massage and are quite addictive!

Pillows

Pillows are used for comfortable positioning. I recommend using standard-size bed pillows.

Towels

If you're using oil, you'll need a towel to clean up oil drips. Keep in mind that oil can stain fabric, so save your fancy towels and use the old ones.

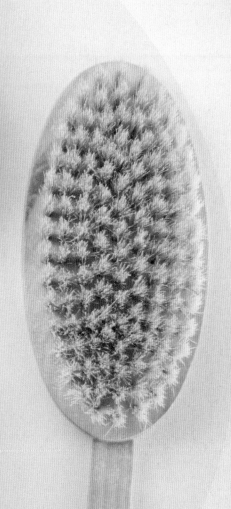

touch

is the

first sense

your body

develops

A Few Things to Keep in Mind Before Beginning

1. Wash your hands with soap and water. Besides being hygienic, this clears away negative energy.
2. Remove any jewelry that may get in the way (i.e., rings that may scratch, bracelets that dangle).
3. Create a comfortable environment with regard to sounds (play soft, soothing music), lighting (dim lights are preferable), and smells (scented candles or incense can help set the mood).
4. Make sure you have everything you need (oil, lotion, towel) in reach and position yourself comfortably.
5. Ground yourself by taking your shoes off (so you feel the floor).
6. Center yourself by closing your eyes and picturing a warm golden light around yourself and the person you will be touching. This calms your energy and focuses your attention. Rub your palms together to get the energy flowing and warm your hands.
7. Always communicate with the person you are going to touch and, when you touch them, ask how it feels.
8. Take a few deep breaths and relax.

TOUCH THERAPIES
ARE "HOLISTIC": THEY CONSIDER
THE WHOLE PERSON—BODY, MIND,
SPIRIT, AND EMOTIONS—IN THE
QUEST FOR OPTIMAL HEALTH
AND WELLNESS.

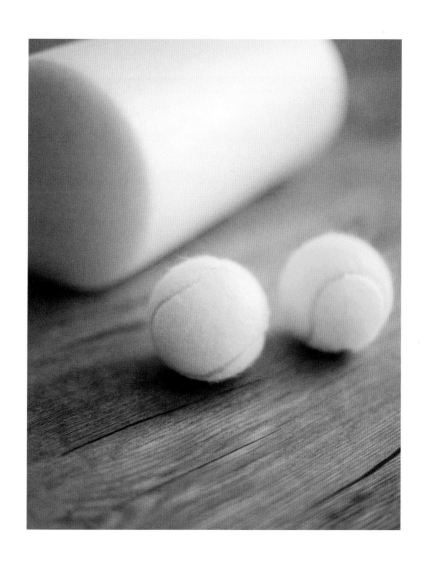

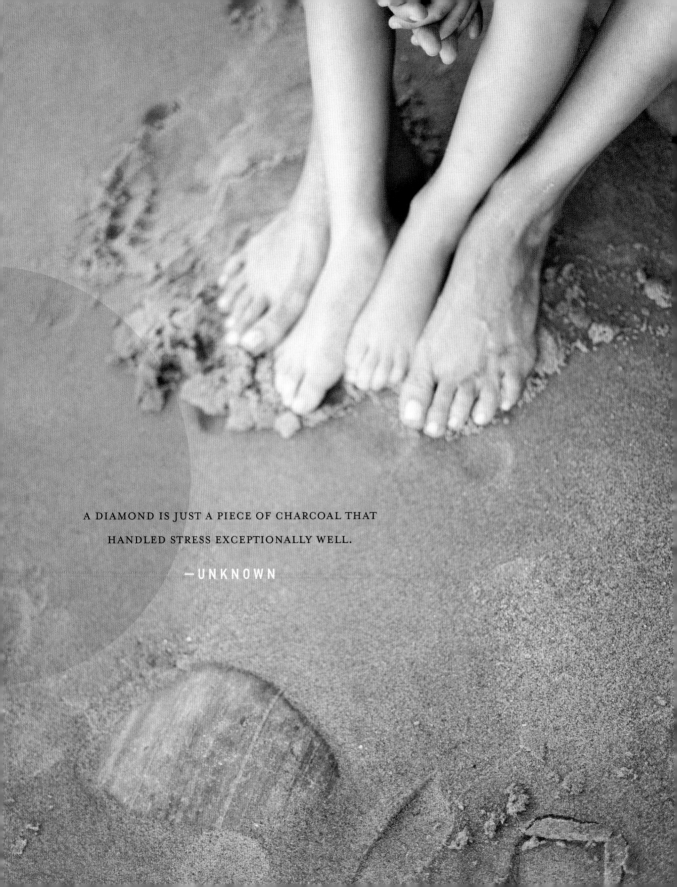

A DIAMOND IS JUST A PIECE OF CHARCOAL THAT
HANDLED STRESS EXCEPTIONALLY WELL.

—UNKNOWN

CHAPTER TWO

Touch More, Stress Less

The Stress–Touch Connection

As a massage therapist and business owner for over twenty years as well as a mother of three boys, I've certainly encountered my share of stressed-out men and women of all ages. And all of them have been more than willing to voice how the pressures of daily life are wearing them down. "I'm totally stressed!" is something I've heard countless times—and I'm sure most of us are used to hearing (and saying!) it on a daily basis too.

But how many times have you heard someone say, "I'm totally touch deprived"? Not too many, right? Most people are unaware that there's an epidemic of touch deprivation in our culture. This serious lack of touch is adding even more anxiety and stress to our already stress-filled lives. Similar to the way stress can damage your body, a lack of touch can lead to aggression, depression, pain, and many other physical and emotional health problems.[1]

Truth be told, most of us, regardless of our relationship status, are in need of more touch than we're getting. Some of us just don't know it yet. I'm here to tell you that bringing more touch into your life can not only lighten your stress load; it can naturally improve your physical and emotional health, your relationships, and your life. Simply increase the touch factor, and you decrease the stress factor!

Before I go on about all the bad things stress can do to you and all the good things touch can do, I'd like to draw your attention to the touch-versus-stress disparity that's challenging our society today. We live in a fast-paced, technology-driven, touch-phobic society in which the typical daily amount of touch is low and the amount of stress is high. In a study of affluent countries, including Australia, Brazil, Canada, France, Germany, Hong Kong, Italy, Japan, Mexico, and the UK, the United States has one of the highest rates of stress.[2] At the same time, research shows that we touch each other less than people in most other countries.[3] Whether we touch less because we're more stressed or we're more stressed because we touch less is unknown.

Regardless, the combination of high stress and a lack of touch is not healthy. In numerous scientific studies on touch at the University of Miami's Touch Research Institute, Dr. Tiffany Field has demonstrated that living in our largely touch-deprived Western society can have negative consequences, including more stress. This tremendous amount of stress has shaken our nation and caused many people—a whopping ninety-four million to be exact—to rely on anti-anxiety drugs, antidepressants, and other prescription drugs to control some of the physical and emotional symptoms.[4]

Rather than turning to drugs for relief, I'm offering you another option; a real antidote to stress that has been scientifically proven to work—touch therapy. Sure, there are other therapies, such as yoga, meditation, and breathing techniques that can also help reduce your stress. However, touch has an added benefit. Not only is it scientifically proven to decrease the effects of stress; it gives you the ability to communicate a wide range of emotions, which can lead to clear, almost immediate changes in how people think and behave.[5]

By simply touching people you can affect their thoughts and actions. For example, studies found that students who received a supportive touch on their back or arm from a teacher were nearly twice as likely to volunteer in class as those who did not. A caring touch from a doctor left patients with the impression that the visit lasted twice as long, compared with estimates from patients who were untouched. Even professional NBA basketball teams who are "touchier" respond by performing better on the court! Seriously. In a study at Berkeley led by psychologist Michael W. Kraus, scientists found that NBA teams who touched each other the most during games (and that included every bump, hug, and high five) ranked higher than teams who didn't touch as much. In 2010, the most "touch-bonded" teams were the Boston Celtics and the Los Angeles Lakers, who happened to be two of the league's top teams. As for individual players, the touchiest was Kevin Garnett, the Celtics' star player, who reached out and touched four other players, just 600 milliseconds after shooting a free throw![6]

Although some people are naturally "touchier" than others, touch benefits everyone. Touch helps givers feel closer to the people they touch, and it helps receivers feel closer to those who touch them. Now, it's not clear which comes first, the touching or the feeling of closeness. In other words, we don't know if people touch one other because they already feel close to them, or they feel close to people because they have touched them. However, one usually leads to the other and, as numerous studies have established, touch produces advantageous results.

In addition to being a great stress reliever, touch is a vital means of emotional expression. The gentle touch of someone's caring hand can lift you up when you're feeling down, soothe your nerves when you're feeling tense, and strengthen all of your relationships.[7] Touch can help you relax and intimately connect with someone at the same time. "Touch may even be stronger than words, gestures, or expressions in many circumstances," according to Dr. Tiffany Field.[8] For example, a mother's hand on her child's feverish forehead can calm her child more than words, just as a friend's sympathetic shoulder squeeze or a partner's loving embrace can convey so much more than words alone.

In some instances, such as personal tragedies like prolonged illness or death, when there are no words to say, touch is the only way to express how you feel. According to Dacher Keltner, professor of psychology at the University of California, Berkeley, "Whether it's a pat on your shoulder, an enthusiastic high five, a momentary touch, or the extensive touch from a professional massage, touch is an ideal way to spread goodness to others."[9] And that's not a bad thing in this day and age, when being so ultraconnected through technology has left so many of us feeling disconnected.

Over the years I've witnessed tremendous transformations take place in individuals and families when touch therapies are used on a regular basis. Scientific studies prove that touch has the power to counteract many of the negative effects of stress. Not only does it decrease levels of cortisol, the

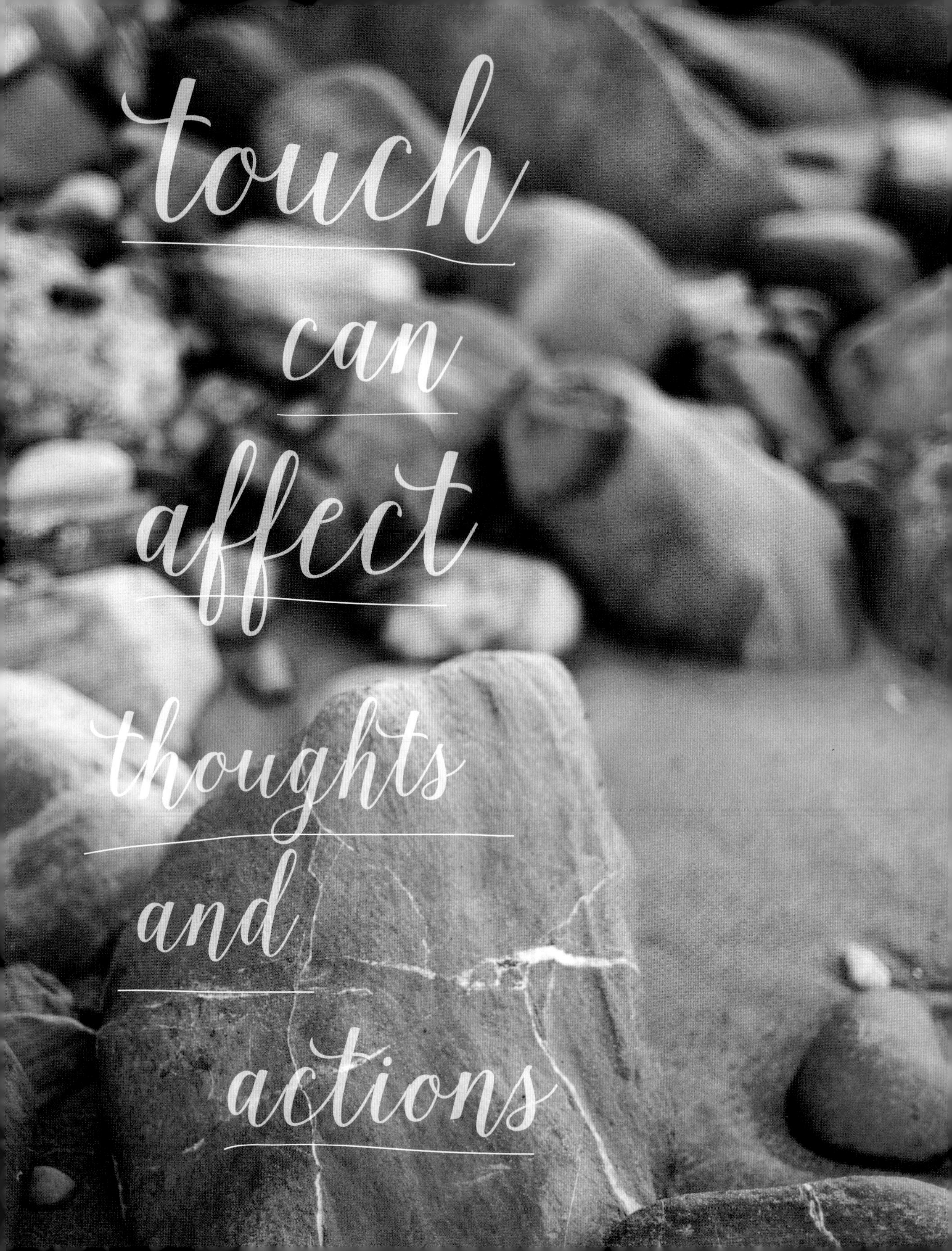

touch

can

affect

thoughts

and

actions

body's stress hormone; it's even more beneficial than receiving social support, such as someone to talk to or a shoulder to cry on, from family or friends. Throughout this book I'll disclose many personal tales of how touch transformed people close to me. But anecdotal stories have never been enough for me. I've always needed concrete evidence to convince me to try something. After many years of examining studies on how stress affects the body as well as researching how different touch therapies can relieve stress-related problems, practicing the techniques on hundreds of people, and getting clients' feedback, I can tell you one thing for sure: *touch therapy works!*

Before we begin the specific touch remedies, it's important that you learn the facts on the real effects of stress. It may scare you a little, but I hope it will also motivate you to take an honest look at the stress in your life and the necessary steps to overcome it. After you're sufficiently alarmed by the "stressful" data, I'll share some of the amazing scientific studies from research centers all over the world that prove how touch can work wonders, even change your brain chemistry, and how different forms of touch therapy can positively improve your health.

All this is meant to inspire you to take care of yourself and your family by giving touch a try. All of the touch remedies, with the exception of a few partner techniques, can be done on yourself. You can also do them to the members of your family, so everyone can experience the benefits of touch. No matter who you are, how young or old, touch can change your life! With nothing but your own two hands and some basic knowledge, you really can overcome stress and get rid of the harmful symptoms it causes in your own body and in those you care about.

Stress

Whether it's work, the kids, finances, or the car alarm going off down the street, stress is inevitable, and everyone encounters some form of it on a daily basis. Stress can affect your health, relationships, career, and overall quality of life.

Not too long ago, stress was considered a problem that mostly occurred after a life crisis such as a death, serious illness, divorce, unemployment, or other traumatic event. Today, however, advances in technology (such as the cell phone that's permanently stuck to everyone's hand) have enabled us to constantly multitask, absorb different streams of media (e-mail, TV, social media, etc.) at once, and take on ever more projects and responsibilities. According to the *New York Times,* Americans today take in more than three times as much data as they did in 1960.[10] However, all of this advancing technology isn't just making us more productive. New evidence shows that it's making us more stressed and less discerning about how much and what kind of information we absorb.[11] Maybe our brains really aren't supposed to process this much random data after all.

This information overload has led to widespread chronic stress that exists both externally, with the pressures around us, and internally, in how we handle those pressures. External stress, such as work deadlines, finances, or personal and professional relationship problems, is tangible. Internal stress, on the other hand, shows itself as the subtle, and sometimes not so subtle, symptoms with which the body signals that you're out of balance, compromising your mental, emotional, and physical health and exhausting your energy supply faster than you can replenish it. Stress is actually defined as "a perception of a real or imagined threat to your body or your ego."[12] So whether the stress you perceive is real (a war, for example) or imagined (say, fear of losing your job), the perception itself creates the same response in the body, regardless of its origin.

Today, the duration and persistency of stress has made it a silent killer.[13] As economic pressures become greater than ever before and it becomes harder to turn off the barrage of information streaming at us, it also becomes harder to buffer ourselves from the world. As we race through our days on constant "high alert," not giving our bodies time to relax and recharge between what our minds perceive as "crises," stress hormones build up and begin to damage our bodies. (A crisis, by the way, could be something as simple as forgetting something at work or seeing a horrible car crash on TV.) In addition to not getting enough sleep or exercise, our unhealthy, caffeine-fueled diets combined with the 24/7 news cycle further impair our ability to recuperate from stress. No wonder we're in a universal state of tension!

As a direct result of our overstimulated, overextended modern lifestyle, we experience a new kind of stress these days called superstress, which resembles—both physically and emotionally—posttraumatic stress disorder (PTSD), according to Roberta Lee, author of *The SuperStress Solution*.[14] Superstress occurs when your body is continually in a "stress response" state and rarely, if ever, gets to rejuvenate with a "relaxation response." If you've ever felt physically and emotionally exhausted by continually struggling to keep up with all the demands in your life and you feel as though you're losing perspective on what's important, you are probably feeling some of the effects of superstress.

Unfortunately, in the accelerated pace of modern life, more and more people have resigned themselves to these increasingly high levels of stress.

According to a survey by the American Psychological Association (APA), 73 percent of all parents report family responsibilities as a significant source of stress, 80 percent of workers feel stressed by their job, and 42 percent of adults say that their stress levels have increased in the past five years. On an average day, one million Americans call in sick for stress-related reasons.[15] The Centers for Disease Control and Prevention (CDC) report that stress is the single highest cause of worker absenteeism, double that of all other illnesses and injuries.[16] Apparently, workplace stress is as bad for your heart as smoking and high cholesterol![17] In fact, over 70 percent of all visits to primary care physicians involve stress-related complaints,[18] which include various gastrointestinal, cardiovascular, respiratory, musculoskeletal, skin, psychological, and reproductive disorders.

Since employees with high stress have 46 percent higher health-care costs,[19] and it's well established that stress interferes with memory, concentration, judgment, and decision making, some forward-thinking companies are actually including programs such as yoga, meditation, and massage (yeah!) to help manage the amount of stress employees experience in the workplace. This is an exciting trend, and I look forward to more companies expanding their preventative health programs. As study after study has found that workers under emotional stress are less productive and less engaged,[20] more in-office programs to encourage regular stress relief will benefit both employers and employees.

What's disconcerting is the fact that some people actually believe that stress makes them more productive. Most people just aren't conscious of the full impact stress is having on them. So instead of addressing their stress and finding ways to minimize it, they end up focusing on the ailments and diseases caused by it. Persistent long-term stress can do great harm to your body, and it's essential that you understand exactly what that means, so you can make sure it doesn't happen to you!

NO MATTER WHO YOU ARE, HOW YOUNG OR OLD, TOUCH CAN CHANGE YOUR LIFE.

Effects of Stress

Stress . . . anxiety, frustration, impatience, inability to focus, bitchiness! Stress not only affects your body; it dramatically affects your emotions and alters the way you think, act, and feel. And nothing ages you faster, internally and externally, than high stress. Yet although I've focused on all the negative effects of stress, it's important to note that stress is part of the human condition and is actually necessary to a degree. In fact, stress and fear are essential for human survival. Stress hormones help you become alert and aware, so you can react quickly in any situation. They can help you raise levels of performance (ace that tennis match!), pursue challenging goals (rock that business meeting!), and, primitively, help you respond to perceived dangers by triggering your fight-or-flight instinct with a boost of adrenaline when you need it most.

Cortisol, the primary stress hormone, which many people consider "bad" for the body, is actually necessary in small doses. It's produced when you first wake up in the morning and is one of the hormones responsible for helping you get rid of brain fog and invigorating your brain and body to "turn on." Researchers say that there's an anxiety "sweet spot," an optimal level of stress that lies somewhere between checked out and freaked out, in which a person is motivated to succeed, yet not so anxious that performance takes a dive.[21] Yet, although a little stress and small amounts of stress hormones can benefit you on occasion, long-lasting stress can be toxic and extremely damaging to your body and mind; it can also exacerbate existing health problems.

It's important to recognize that there are two types of stress: stress that affects you suddenly (acute short-term stress) and stress that affects you over time (chronic long-term stress). Acute stress—any situation that seems demanding or dangerous, such as someone grabbing your bag on the street or a dog surprising you with an angry bark—causes your body to respond instantly. It then normally recovers fairly quickly. Acute stress can cause problems, however, if it happens too often or if you don't have a chance to recover. Chronic stress, on the other hand, is more damaging, because it's caused by stressful situations or events that last over a long period of time, such as a difficult job or a chronic disease. To fully realize just how damaging stress can be to your body and mind, it's important to understand exactly what happens to you in response to both acute and chronic stress.

Acute Stress

Say, for example, out of the blue you hear a loud explosion. Here's what happens. First, a part of your brain called the hypothalamic-pituitary-adrenal

(HPA) system is activated, which triggers the release of stress hormones, called neurotransmitters, including norepinephrine, adrenaline, and cortisol. These neurotransmitters activate an area inside your brain called the amygdala, which appears to trigger your emotional response, such as fear or anxiety, to a stressful event. This also triggers the fight-or-flight response, causing your heart rate and blood pressure to increase and your muscles to contract. All of this happens in a split second and is beyond your control.

But that's not all. When you're stressed, your brain releases a small protein called neuropeptide S, which increases alertness and your sense of anxiety (so that you can respond quickly to problems) and decreases sleep (that's why you have insomnia and continually wake up during the night when you're stressed). The neurotransmitters also mess with your brain by suppressing activity in the front of the brain, the area concerned with memory, concentration, inhibition, and rational thought. So although stress may help you react quickly to perceived dangers, your ability to think straight and remember things during those stress-filled moments can be slightly to profoundly impaired.

At the same time your brain is activated, your body snaps into action with an instantaneous increase in heart rate and blood pressure. Your breathing becomes shallow and fast, and your lungs take in more oxygen. When you're superstressed, your blood flow can actually increase 300 to 400 percent to prepare your muscles, lungs, and brain for a potential challenge. As fluids are diverted from a nonessential location such as your mouth, you can experience dry mouth as well as difficulty talking and swallowing. Blood flows away from the skin to support the heart and muscles, causing clammy hands and sweaty armpits. Your digestive system shuts down, so you're left with an upset stomach, nausea, or diarrhea, and your immune system is weakened. In addition, a headache, a stiff neck, tight shoulders, and back pain often accompany all of these common symptoms. Sound familiar?

However, the good news is that under most circumstances, once the stressful event is over, levels of stress hormones return to normal, and many of these symptoms disappear. This is called the "relaxation response."[22]

Chronic Stress

If stress is persistent and your body never has the chance to arrive at the "relaxation response," stress becomes chronic and can damage you physically and psychologically. Your body responds to chronic stress primitively. For our ancestors thousands of years ago, long-term stress meant the threat of not having enough to eat. Consequently, our innate physiological response to chronic stress developed to prepare our bodies for famine. The natural secretion of cortisol, the stress hormone, causes our metabolism to begin burning proteins, including connective tissue, fascia, and muscle tissue. Recent studies have linked increased cortisol in the body to increases in appetite and cravings for foods high in sugar and fat as well as more storage of fat, especially in the abdomen.[23] And no one needs that! Since our bodies don't know the difference between a physical threat, like a famine, and an abstract threat, such as a work or relationship problem, we respond in the same way we did thousands of years ago, and chronic stress begins.[24] In a state of chronic stress, stress hormones never return to normal levels, and you begin to develop additional stress-related symptoms.

Today, studies link chronic stress to the development and worsening of many medical conditions, including:

- High blood pressure and heart disease
- Diabetes and cancer
- Weakened immune system
- Muscle and joint pain (specifically neck, shoulder, and back pain)
- Gastrointestinal problems (including ulcers, irritable bowel syndrome, colitis, diarrhea, constipation, cramping, and bloating)
- PMS
- Chronic fatigue syndrome
- Insomnia and sleep disorders
- Sexual problems and low fertility
- Autoimmune and inflammatory diseases
- Fibromyalgia
- Asthma
- Skin problems (acne and psoriasis)
- Migraines
- Rheumatoid arthritis
- Eating disorders and weight gain and obesity
- Depression and anxiety
- Lack of concentration and memory problems
- Unexplained hair loss (alopecia)
- Periodontal disease
- Substance abuse
- For pregnant women, a higher risk for miscarriage, lower infant birth weight, and an increased incidence of premature births; for infants, a higher rate of crying and low attention[25]

Watch Out, Stress Is Contagious!

In addition to all of these serious physical problems, stress is contagious. Whether it's at home or the office, new studies suggests that stress transfers from one person to another.[26] Researchers found that just being around a stressed person, whether a loved one or a stranger, has the power to make you stressed in a physically quantifiable way. Simply observing a person in a stressful situation, whether in person or on a video, can be enough to make your own body release the stress hormone cortisol.[27] Rather than just feeling sympathetic for a coworker or partner who's stressed out, you actually take on some of that person's stress and your own body reacts as if you are under stress.

There's "crossover stress" between spouses and between coworkers, and "spillover stress" from the work to the home. Referred to as the 'stress contagion effect,' it spreads anxiety like a virus wreaking havoc on not just you, but everyone around you. In fact, if your partner is stressed, you're 25 percent more likely to be affected than a stranger would be.[28] And that can be hard on your relationships and your health! As the researchers noted, "In our stress-ridden society, empathic stress is a phenomenon that should not be ignored by the health-care system."[29]

In a nutshell, stress reduces your quality of life all around. It can harm your body and mind and put a damper on your feelings of pleasure, accomplishment, and above all happiness. So it makes sense to do everything in your power to decrease the stress in your life. How can we do that? I suggest touch.

Touch

We Are Touch Hungry

In today's "plugged-in" society, you would think that people would be more connected to one another than ever before as a result of online social networking (thank you, Facebook), texting, and technology that follows us everywhere, even to the top of a mountain. However, nothing could be farther from the truth. In reality, people are lonelier and more distant and disconnected from one another.[30] A lack of intimacy is straining all of our relationships, and touch is a crucial component of intimacy. Touch is as critical for adults' physical and mental well-being as it is for children's growth, development, and health. Whether you realize it or not, it's a fundamental part of our daily experience, influencing what we buy, who we love, and even how we heal. We use it to gather information about our surroundings and as a means

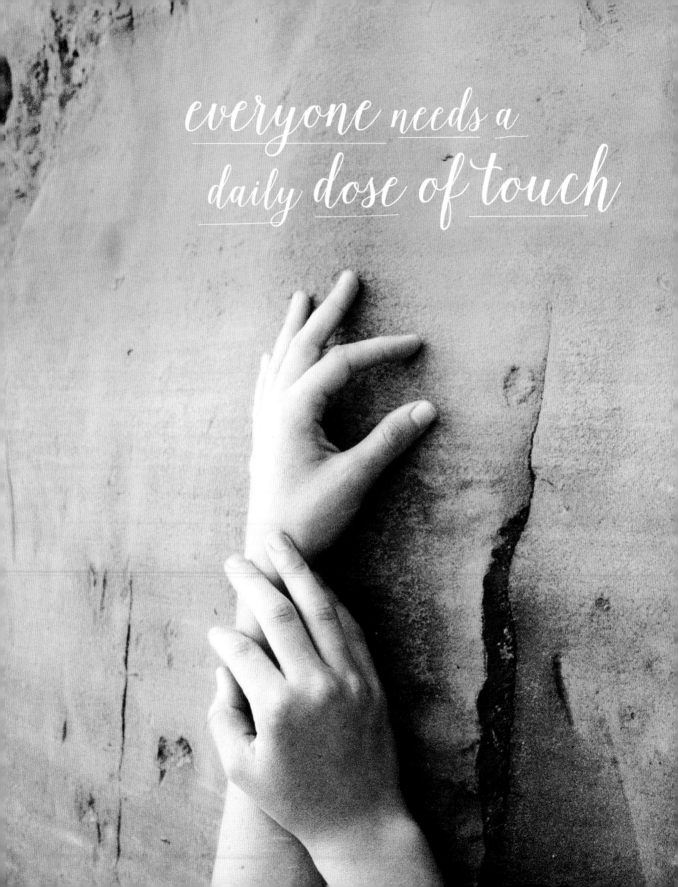

of establishing trust and social bonds with other people.[31] Unfortunately, we're just not getting enough of it.

Nowadays many people are "dangerously touch deprived" and suffer from "touch hunger," according to Tiffany Field, the pioneer researcher on touch at Miami's Touch Research Institute.[32] This is a real problem that we shouldn't ignore, because it can lead to harmful stress-related problems such as lack of energy, anxiety, self-destructive behavior, sexual problems, a sense of isolation, and much more. According to psychology professor David R. Cross, at Texas Christian University, "Humans deprived of touch are prone to mental illness, violence, compromised immune systems, and poor self-regulation."[33] So serious are the effects of touch deprivation, it's considered by researchers to be worse than physical abuse during early childhood.[34] Unfortunately, although there is scientific research proving that a lack of touch is detrimental to health, because the effects are more insidious and long-term, they haven't yet provoked urgent concern by the general public or health officials.

In the United States, we have one of the lowest rates of casual touch in the world. Compared to other cultures where double-cheek kisses and hugs are standard greetings, Americans are hesitant to touch each other (even the traditional handshake is slowly being replaced by the fist bump), and we like to keep our distance from others. Unlike most of the world, where people are comfortable with 1 to 2 feet of personal space between them, most Americans need 2 to 4 feet of personal space to feel comfortable.[35] In a well-known study comparing how many times couples from different countries touched each other while sitting at a café, researchers found that in Mexico City couples touched each other 185 times, in Paris 115 times, and in Gainesville, Florida, only twice.[36]

In fact, "touchier" countries have an advantage. Studies show that cultures in which there is more physically affectionate touch toward infants and children, such as France, have less aggression and lower rates of adult violence.[37] In one study, scientists compared the way parents touched their small children on playgrounds in Paris and Miami and how adolescents touched each other in McDonald's in those same cities. They found that the French children, who received more physical affection from their parents, were less physically and verbally aggressive toward their peers on the playground than the children in Miami. The French adolescents were also more physically affectionate toward each other and showed less verbal and physical aggression.[38] Research by neuropsychologist James W. Prescott indicates that insufficient amounts of physical affection may be a cause of high violence rates in the United States.[39] This is a great incentive for all of us to increase the amount of touch in our families today.

Why Don't We Touch Each Other?

According to Dr. Cross, there are three main reasons Americans don't touch each other more: fear of sexual innuendo, societal and personal disconnection aided by technology, and the fact that the ill effects of non-touching are simply not that obvious and don't receive much attention.[40] (This is one reason I wrote this book!) Believe it or not, in the early 1950s, parenting manuals advised parents not to touch their children too much—recommending that, instead of hugs and kisses, parents give kids a "pat on the head."[41] Parents were encouraged not to shower their children with affection, as this would make them weak and unprepared for the world.

There are many more cultural taboos, mostly unspoken and mainly regarding sex, that have led us to be touch hungry. For sure, in our oversexualized society there's a tendency to sexualize all physical contact.[42] As a result, most touching between people is reserved for spouses or significant others and close family. Many parents are uncomfortable touching their own children, especially of the opposite sex and particularly when they are approaching adolescence, for fear that it may be misconstrued as sexually inappropriate. And although it's slowly becoming more acceptable, it's still rare to see same-sex couples holding hands in public.

There's a taboo against touch at schools, where teachers are instructed not to touch their students and antitouch laws have been put into place. Teachers in some schools now are no longer allowed to hug grade-schoolers if they do well in class or pick up preschoolers when they fall on the playground.[43] On an Oprah Winfrey show that focused on the issue of teachers touching children, the president of the National Education Association even said, "Our slogan is, 'Teach. Don't touch.'"

Some of the other fear-based taboos against touch in our culture that have led us to be touch hungry include:

"Don't touch the opposite gender!"—based on the belief that all touch is sexual.

"Don't touch same-gender friends!"—based on homophobic fears.

"Don't touch yourself!"—based on religious and puritanical doctrines and fears.

"Don't touch strangers!"—based on a cultural fear of those who are outside of one's own group.

"Don't touch the elderly, the sick, or the dying!"—based on fear, lack of knowledge, and the negative attitude in our culture that segregates the elderly, the sick, and the dying from the rest of the population.[44]

There are so many both conscious and subconscious reasons why we hold back from touching each other and ourselves. It's really no wonder, then, that we're all craving touch, whether we know it or not. Even if you think you're getting enough touch every day, you probably don't realize how much better you'd feel if you got just a little more.

Touch Is Key

The importance of touch cannot be overestimated. Touch is essential to our physical and mental vitality, and, like diet and exercise, everybody needs a daily dose of it. Referred to as the "mother of all senses," touch is the first sense to develop in the womb and the first language we learn.[45] It's ten times more communicative than verbal contact, and it affects everything we do.[46] Neuroscientist David Linden argues that the "genes, cells, and neural circuits involved in the sense of touch have been crucial to creating our unique human experience."[47] We take in and process physical, social, and emotional information about our environment through touch. And according to psychologist Dacher Keltner, "Touch . . . is the primary language of compassion, love and gratitude—emotions at the heart of trust and cooperation."[48] Research by DePauw University psychologist Matthew Hertenstein shows that touch can communicate multiple emotions, including joy, love, gratitude, and sympathy.[49]

Touch Is Win-Win

One of the best things about touch is that it doesn't matter if you're the giver or the recipient; you both benefit. "The more you connect with others—on even the smallest physical level—the happier you'll be," explains neurologist

YOU HAVE THE POWER IN YOUR HANDS TO PROVIDE IMMEDIATE REWARDS AND FOSTER TRUST AND GENEROSITY IN ANYONE, ANYTIME, SIMPLY THROUGH TOUCH.

Shekar Raman, based in Richmond, Virginia.[50] Touch works both ways, because your brain processes the stimulation from the nerve endings under your skin whether you're touching or being touched.

According to Edmund Rolls, a psychologist and neuroscientist at Cambridge University, the orbitofrontal cortex (OFC) is the part of our brain that helps us navigate our physical and social environments and helps us bring about more rewarding social encounters.[51] He documented that our brains perceive touch, whether we're giving or getting it, as a reward. For example, scientists have found that depressed mothers who are encouraged to touch and massage their infants regularly experience reduced symptoms of depression and begin to play more with their children. Elderly individuals who volunteer to give massages to infants report reductions in their own anxiety and depression and enhanced well-being.[52]

Touch triggers the brain's reward center, but it also fosters trust and generosity. For instance, in one study, participants were asked to sign a petition in support of a particular issue of local importance. Those participants who were touched signed 81 percent of the time. Those who were not touched signed 55 percent of the time.[53] Here are a few more research-supported examples:

> Customers respond more positively to a supermarket taste test and purchase request when touched by a store assistant.
>
> Individuals who have been touched are more likely to agree to participate in mall interviews.
>
> People are significantly more likely to return a coin left in a phone booth if the preceding "telephone caller" touched them.[54]

The good news is that *you* have the power in your hands to provide immediate rewards (pleasure) and foster trust and generosity in anyone, anytime, simply through touch. If even the briefest touch can elicit strong emotional experiences, just imagine how beneficial thoughtful, purpose-driven, nurturing touch can be.

How Touch Works

Our skin is our largest organ—adults carry about 8 pounds of it covering approximately 22 square feet—and biologically it's our first line of defense against infections and disease. Our skin, when we are touching or receiving touch, is a pathway to comfort and healing. But there is also a lot happening *under* the skin that scientists are just beginning to understand. Extensive research indicates that skin-to-skin touch triggers a real physiological reaction in the body, one that is the opposite of the stress reaction. When you're touched, receptors under the skin, called C-fibers (also known as "caress sensors"), are stimulated, and two pathways in the brain are triggered. The first is a sensory pathway, which gives us the facts about touch, like vibration, pressure, location, and texture. The second pathway processes social and emotional information, determining the emotional content of the touch. This second pathway activates brain regions associated with social bonding and pleasure and pain centers.[55]

Here's how it works in the brain. The orbitofrontal cortex (OFC—the part of your brain involved in decision making and also linked to feelings of reward and compassion) is *activated,* while the hypothalamic-pituitary-adrenal (HPA) axis, which responds to stress, is *deactivated.* A cascade of chemical responses occurs, including a decrease in stress hormones (cortisol, catecholamines, norepinephrine, epinephrine) and an increase in oxytocin (the "love hormone," which promotes feelings of devotion and trust), serotonin, and dopamine (the body's "happiness" chemicals and natural sources of pleasure and pain relief). The shift in these biochemicals has been proven to calm the nervous system, balance your heart rate, lower blood pressure, strengthen the body's immune system, and reduce depression, pain, and anxiety.[56] These feel-good chemicals also trigger the activation of the vagus nerve, the nerve bundle in the body associated with promoting feelings of trust and social connection.[57]

Touch also *deactivates* the amygdala, which, if you'll remember from my earlier explanation of stress, is the part of the brain that triggers emotional responses, such as fear or anxiety, and is *activated* by stress.[58] Thus, in many ways, touch is an antidote to stress. Interestingly, in our touch-deprived world people subconsciously turn to things like pedicures, haircuts, and even contact football and basketball games for ways to trigger activation in the orbitofrontal cortex and the release of these calming biochemicals.[59]

Everyone needs touch to thrive, especially babies. "If you don't get touch right after you're born, all kinds of terrible things happen, and not just cognitive and emotional ones," states Dr. Linden. "Your immune system doesn't develop properly, your digestive system tends to have problems—there's a whole rack of health problems that can develop if you don't receive touch in early life."[60]

Some of you may remember the shocking reports on Romanian orphanages that leaked to the West after the fall of Communism in 1989. In 1990, ABC's *20/20* ran a full exposé revealing the devastating lives of the babies in these overpopulated orphanages, where infant mortality rates rose to 30 to 40 percent. Because of overcrowding and poor resources, these babies went almost entirely untouched. The children were so touch starved that they failed to grow to half their expected height or weight and failed to develop normal cognitive and motor skills. These orphans were found to have diminished growth hormone, and researchers determined that touch deprivation delayed their growth.[61] This was a shocking global awakening to the importance of touch in infancy and early childhood.

Today we know that touch is essential to infants' healthy development. Additional studies have revealed more about the physiological benefits of touch for infants and children. In studies by Tiffany Field at the Touch Research Institute, scientists found that premature infants who were massaged for 15 minutes three times a day gained 47 percent more weight and had faster neurological development than babies who were not massaged.[62] Babies who were massaged also cried less. In a study of children with ADHD, after receiving massage therapy, their aversion to touch, attention to sounds, and off-task classroom behavior decreased while connections to their teachers increased.[63]

For adults, studies published by the National Institutes of Health (NIH) show that massage therapy has tremendous benefits. Massage therapy can:

- Alleviate lower-back pain and improve range of motion
- Improve the condition of the body's largest organ—the skin
- Increase joint flexibility
- Lessen depression and anxiety
- Improve sleep by increasing delta waves in the brain
- Relieve migraine and headache pain
- Relax and soften injured, tired, and overused muscles
- Release endorphins—amino acids that work as the body's natural painkillers

- Pump oxygen and nutrients into tissues and vital organs, improving circulation
- Enhance immunity by stimulating lymph flow—the body's natural defense system
- Ease medication dependence
- Exercise and stretch weak, tight, or atrophied muscles
- Help athletes of any level prepare for and recover from strenuous workouts
- Promote tissue regeneration, reducing scar tissue and stretch marks
- Reduce postsurgery adhesions and swelling
- Reduce spasms and cramping
- Assist with shorter, easier labor for expectant mothers and shorten maternity hospital stays[64]

Further scientific studies by the Touch Research Institute on adults, children, and babies prove that massage can help the additional following problems:

- Arthritis
- Asthma
- Autism
- High blood pressure
- Burns
- Cerebral palsy
- Eating disorders: anorexia and bulimia
- Fibromyalgia
- Diabetes
- Digestive disorders
- Menopausal symptoms
- Multiple sclerosis (MS)
- Myofascial pain syndrome and nerve pain
- Premenstrual syndrome (PMS)
- Posttraumatic stress disorder (PTSD)
- Pregnancy-related issues
- Soft tissue muscle strains or injuries
- Temporomandibular joint disorders (TMJ and TMD)[65]

Stress Management

Now that I've explained how touch can help you combat many of the harmful effects of stress, it's time to put touch to work for you. Stress will always be out there, but you don't have to be held captive by it. You can escape stress by controlling your response to it and thus manage it from the inside out. That means understanding *when* your body and mind are experiencing all the big and little "stress responses" throughout the day. And then give yourself permission to take the time to allow the "relaxation response" to happen— even if it's just a 5-minute break in your day. When you can identify the instances when you're stressed and then put into practice stress-management techniques like the touch-therapy remedies in this book, you'll find that your stress level decreases and you feel more in control.

Stress management is a powerful tool for wellness—and it's crucial to your health that you learn to cope with stress in positive ways. "What am I doing to take care of myself today?" is a question you should ask yourself on a daily basis. By managing stress in healthy ways you not only promote better health and happiness for yourself, but if you are a parent, you also promote the formation of critically important habits and skills in your children.[66]

The touch-therapy remedies in this book will help you manage the stress in your life. They can reduce anxiety, give you more energy, help you sleep better, improve your concentration, reduce fatigue, and improve your overall well-being. Getting a professional massage regularly is unrealistic for most people, but these effective self-care remedies offer a sensible, cost-free way for you to experience the benefits of touch whenever you need them!

In a world in which stress just doesn't go away, I encourage you to take a few minutes to bring some calm into your otherwise hectic day and use touch remedies to live more healthfully. In the following chapters, I'll give you all the scientific evidence for each touch remedy and explain how to use touch to enhance your health during specific times in your life. My goal is to motivate you to take control of your health and use the power of touch to improve your life and the lives of everyone you care about. Let the touch revolution begin!

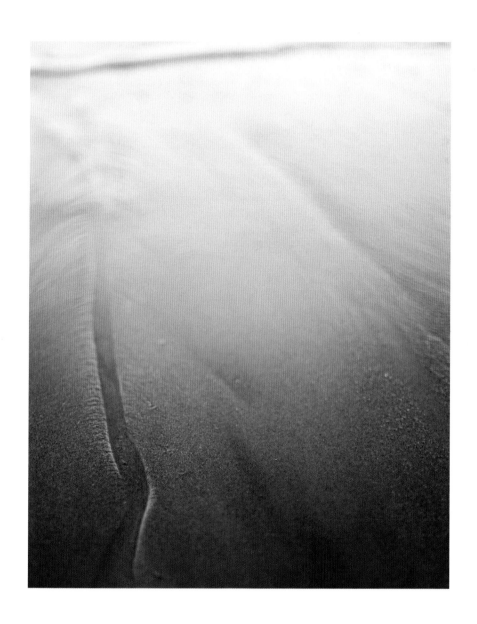

THE BODY IS PRECIOUS. IT IS OUR VEHICLE FOR AWAKENING. TREAT IT WITH CARE.

—BUDDHA

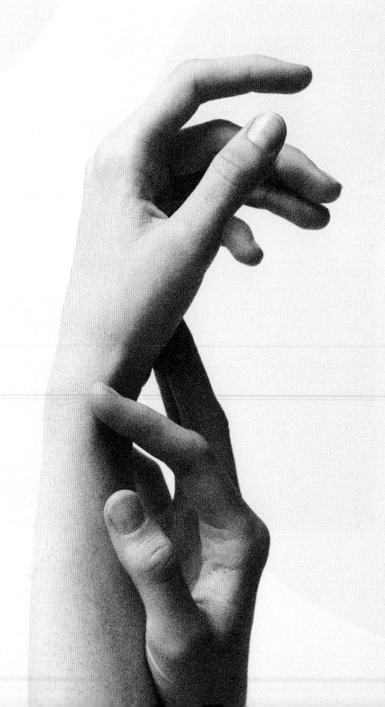

CHAPTER THREE

Hands on You

DIY Self-Care for Every Body

When I'm stressed-out, the last thing I want to do at the end of the day is work out, or make a healthy dinner, or talk to anyone. Really, all I want to do is pour myself a glass of wine and crash in front of the TV. So it's no wonder to me that in today's plugged-in "24-hour society," in which everyone leads an incredibly hectic lifestyle, self-care is often the first thing to go when stress kicks in. When we're stressed, our brains go into fight-or-flight mode, and our perspective on how to cope with stress narrows.[1] It happens to everyone! Rather than pay attention to how stress is affecting us and actually do something about it, we either ignore it or complain about it and procrastinate in doing anything to remedy the situation. In both cases, we neglect ourselves and end up suffering physically and mentally.

No more excuses. You don't have to be a prisoner of stress anymore!

You can, and must, take care of yourself every single day. My DIY touch remedies are easy to learn, and you can use them anywhere, anytime. At work, they're great when you need to give yourself a break to jump-start your body's "relaxation response" and avoid the typical "stress response." The remedies can enhance your body awareness and bring a sense of calm by encouraging you to tune out what's going on around you and tune into what you're feeling inside. By slowing down and focusing on what you're feeling physically and emotionally, you can connect to the place of stillness and peace that exists in everyone. After reading this chapter, you won't need anything other than your own two hands to help you relieve many of the physical and emotional problems caused by the pressures of daily life.

Although you can't control the circumstances that life throws your way, you can control how you react to them and how you take care of yourself. Stress is unavoidable, so it's essential that you find ways to deal with it before it takes over your life. Managing stress doesn't have to be about making huge lifestyle changes or rethinking your career goals, but rather learning how to make self-care a priority. No, I'm not suggesting that everyone must get a professional massage regularly (although that's not a bad thing). Instead, I'm suggesting a more realistic life adjustment—to be proactive and do something simple every day to take care of *yourself.*

Self-care should become a habit, so that when you're feeling stressed you automatically think, "Hey, I need to take care of myself in this situation." Self-care should also be considered a form of self-love. In Ayurvedic medicine, there's a self-massage practice called Abhyanga Sneha; *sneha* can be translated as both "oil" and "love." Self-massage, using any of my touch-therapy remedies, is one of the most beneficial practices you can include in your daily life to enhance your health. More than just making you feel great, it stimulates the lymphatic system, strengthens your immune system, nourishes the skin, reinforces the connection between your body and mind, and calms and rejuvenates the nervous system. Self-massage also teaches you how your touch feels and how differences in pressure feel on different parts of the body, which is very helpful to know when you begin to massage others.

More good news: the benefits of self-care can reach beyond just you. New research reveals that when health-care organizations and their staff engage in self-care as an organizational strategy, it not only improves the healing experience for themselves and patients, but it also improves overall business performance.[2] The research revealed that the health-care system is stressed because the people in it are stressed, and that a fundamental paradigm shift that encourages practicing self-care at home and at work benefits the organization as a whole. According to Dr. Tim Culbert, medical director of Integrative Medicine at Children's Hospital in Minneapolis: "The findings confirm a very basic premise: when people feel better, in all aspects, business measures improve."[3]

I promise, you really don't need anyone else or any drugs to relieve many of the symptoms caused by stress—you can do it yourself. With a little knowledge of touch-therapy techniques you can keep yourself relaxed and healthy. In this chapter, my do-it-yourself touch-therapy remedies provide easy and quick ways to care for your body and mind, to keep you in optimum shape and ready for life's challenges. The touch-therapy remedies include treatments to address:

- Anxiety
- Back pain
- Fatigue and low energy
- Headaches
- Heart disease
- Immunity
- Insomnia
- Weight issues

Use these remedies at home, at work, in the car, standing in line at the store, anywhere. Just use them! And listen to your body—pay attention to what you're feeling and manage your stress with the power of touch.

Anxiety Remedies: "Stress No More"

In our "nervous nation" over the past three decades, anxiety disorders have jumped more than 1,200 percent; as many as 117 million adults in the United States report high levels of anxiety.[4] Come on, who hasn't felt anxious once in a while? When you sense a crisis, anxiety arises in the amygdala, a part of your brain's limbic system that plays a key role in processing emotions. This puts your body on high alert as the amygdala sends impulses to your nervous system that increase heart and breathing rates, tense muscles, and divert blood flow from the abdominal organs to the brain.[5]

Anxiety can actually cause both emotional and *physical* "numbness." Physically, it can lead to anything from tingling to complete lack of feeling, most commonly in the hands, feet, legs, and arms. This is caused by either hyperventilation (breathing too quickly or too shallowly) or overactivation, when blood is directed toward the heart and muscles during a fight-or-flight state. Emotionally, anxiety can lead to the inability to feel emotions, especially positive ones. For example, when people are in shock, they are often unable to react to things, good or bad, because they are emotionally numb.

The following touch-therapy remedies can help you relieve and prevent anxiety quickly. They also provide much-needed tactile stimulation to help restore your equilibrium and bring you back to your senses, so you can literally "feel normal" again.

ANTI-ANXIETY ACUPRESSURE REMEDY

1. *"Third Eye" point:* Using your middle and index fingers, press directly between your eyebrows in the indentation where the bridge of the nose meets the forehead. Press firmly for 10 seconds, release, and repeat several times. Stimulating this point calms the body and relieves nervousness.

2. *"Sea of Tranquility" point:* Place your fourth finger on the center of your breastbone, at the base of the bone. Your index finger should fall directly on the "Sea of Tranquility" point. Press firmly for 10 seconds, release, and repeat several times. This relieves anxiety, chest tension, and nervousness.

3. *"Spirit Gate" point:* Press your thumb on the crease of your wrist, in line with your little finger, on the underside of your forearm. Hold firmly for 10 seconds, release, and repeat. Repeat on your other wrist. Stimulating this point balances emotions and relieves anxiety.

ANTI-ANXIETY REFLEXOLOGY REMEDY

1. *Hand reflex area to the solar plexus:* Press your thumb firmly into the center of your palm. Hold for 10 seconds, release, and then make small circles in one direction for 10 seconds and then 10 seconds in the other. Repeat on the other hand. The solar plexus is the nerve switchboard of the body. Stimulating this spot can balance the nervous system, relieve anxiety, and calm your entire body.

2. *Foot reflex area to the solar plexus:* Press both thumbs directly into the center of the sole of your foot. Hold for 10 seconds, release, and then make small circles in one direction and then the other. Repeat on the other foot.

ANTI-ANXIETY LYMPHATIC MASSAGE REMEDY

A recent study published in the *International Journal of Neuroscience* shows that manual lymphatic-drainage massage is effective in *reducing* the activity of the sympathetic nervous system, which is the part of the autonomic nervous

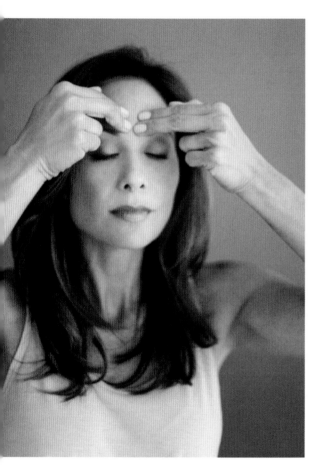

Third Eye Point

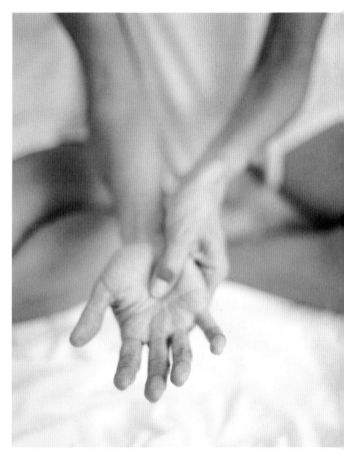

Solar Plexus Reflex Area

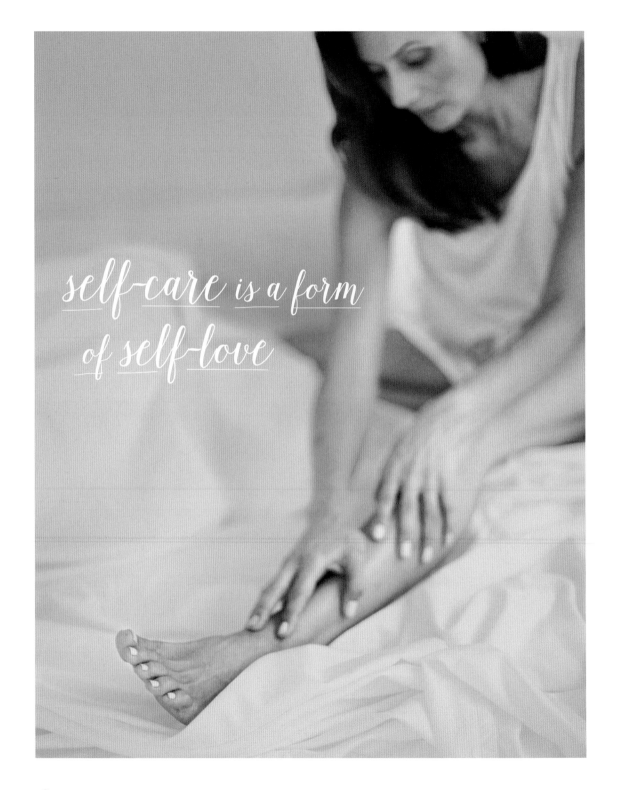

self-care is a form
of self-love

system that reacts under stress with the fight-or-flight response.[6] When you are chronically stressed, the sympathetic nervous system remains active, and this creates an unhealthy state in the body. Lymphatic massage can calm your nervous system and counter stress.

1. Warm some oil or lotion in your hands and, beginning at your feet, stroke upward using a hand-over-hand motion. Apply firm pressure and continue this stroking motion all the way up to your chest. Try to cover your entire body up to chest level, stroking hand over hand upward. This encourages your lymphatic flow to move in the direction of the heart.

2. With one hand, stroke your arm from hand to shoulder. Repeat on the other arm.

3. Finally, switch directions and stroke downward from your neck and shoulders to your heart. Try to touch your entire upper chest area. Always remember to stroke in the direction toward your heart. This soothing self-massage can calm your nerves and keep you mentally and physically balanced.

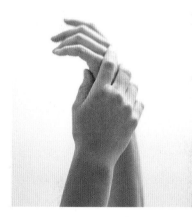

NOTE: *You can also do this with a long-handled, soft-bristled brush, but skip the oil or lotion. I prefer to use a dry brush, because it also exfoliates the skin and I can reach my back and back of my legs easier than with my hands.*

AROMATHERAPY FOR ANXIETY

To enhance the anti-anxiety remedies, mix these oils together and rub a few drops between your fingertips. Inhale the scent and then follow the directions for each remedy. The soothing scent will linger in strategic places on your body.

3 drops lavender oil
4 drops Roman chamomile oil
2 drops clary sage oil
2 drops geranium oil
1 drop ylang ylang oil
2 ounces unscented natural oil

Another option is to add a few drops of vanilla to unscented natural oil. You can use cooking vanilla if you have it handy. In fact, in a 1994 study by Memorial Sloan Kettering Hospital in New York City, patients reported 63 percent less overall anxiety when undergoing MRI scans when the scent of vanilla was present in the room.[7]

ANTI-ANXIETY MEDITATION

One of the things I've found to be extremely helpful in managing anxiety is meditation, which quiets an overactive brain and helps you slow down, get perspective, and think more objectively and with less reactivity. This focused breathing exercise will calm your body and mind and anchor you in the present moment. It's so simple and it only takes a few minutes. Just remember 4-7-8.

1. Inhale through your nose, counting to 4 in your mind (4-second inhalation).

2. With mouth closed, hold your breath and count to 7 in your mind (7-second hold).

3. Exhale through your mouth, counting to 8 in your mind (8-second exhalation).

4. Repeat this cycle four more times.

Back-Pain Remedies: Relieve & Prevent Irritating Backaches

It makes sense that chiropractors and massage therapists everywhere are busy. Over sixty-five million Americans currently suffer from lower-back pain, and it affects 75 percent of the population at some time during their adult lives! It's the second most common reason for medical visits (headaches are number one), the most common cause of job-related disability, and a leading contributor to missed work.[8]

Although most back pain is caused from strain in the muscles that support the spine, it can also be a manifestation of anxiety and stress. Emotional distress often surfaces in the body as chronic back pain. More specifically, emotional stress from relationships can manifest as pain in the middle back, which, interestingly, is directly opposite the heart chakra. There are many theories about the causes of stress-related back pain, including fear of failure, standing up (emotionally and physically) to the demands placed on you, trying to control everything, and an internal conflict of will. In effect, stress-related back pain is caused by various psychological and emotional factors that, together, cause some type of physical change that results in the back pain.

Whether it's caused by emotional stress, lifting a heavy object (like your kid), tripping or falling, pregnancy and labor (I can attest to that), or a viral illness, spasms of the back muscles are painful and debilitating. When spasms are so strong and persistent that they lead to inflammation, a vicious cycle is created that can lead to chronic back, neck, and shoulder pain, migraine headaches, and fatigue. Luckily, nearly 95 percent of lower-back pain can be treated without surgery, and new research proves that massage can help reduce pain and improve mobility and may be an effective short- and longer-term treatment for chronic back pain, with benefits lasting at least six months.[9]

Researchers at the University of Miami School of Medicine conducted a five-week study on people who had been suffering from lower-back pain for at least six months. They found that those who got 30 minutes of massage therapy twice a week had less pain and more mobility and range of motion in their lower back than those who had relaxation therapy during that time.[10] In another study published in the *Scientific World Journal,* researchers investigated whether massage therapy alone for chronic lower-back pain was as effective as combining it with nonsteroid anti-inflammatory drugs. They concluded massage had a positive effect on patients with chronic lower-back pain and proposed that the use of massage causes fast, therapeutic results that could help to reduce the use of anti-inflammatory drugs in the treatment of chronic lower-back pain.[11]

If you're one of the millions of back-pain sufferers, the following reflexology, deep-tissue (rolling-ball), and cranial-sacral remedies can help ease your pain and improve circulation to the spine. Try doing them every day for a week, and you'll notice the results!

BACK-PAIN DEEP-TISSUE REMEDY

1. *Targeting specific areas:* Lie on the floor with your knees bent and feet on the floor. Place a tennis ball under the area where the pain is. If that's too painful, place the tennis ball close to the area. If the sore area is on both sides of the spine, use two tennis balls. (The idea is to relax the muscles around where the pain is to prevent spasms.) The ball should lie on either side of the spine, never directly under it. Gently relax your body weight onto the tennis ball. Next, use your legs to move your body so that the ball rolls a little to massage the area. This can give a fairly deep massage, so move slowly and gently. It should never hurt; rather, it should feel like "aaahh."

2. *Treating the entire spine:* Lie on the floor and place a tennis ball under your lower back on one side of the spine. Keep your knees bent and allow your body weight to relax on the ball. When you're comfortable, use your legs to move your body, so that the ball rolls up the side of the spine, all the way to your neck. Do this very slowly. This improves circulation and relaxes the tight muscles on either side of your spine. Next, move your

body so that the ball rolls back down the spine. Repeat on the other side. This may hurt at first, but if you breathe and move slowly, your muscles will relax and let go.

BACK-PAIN REFLEXOLOGY REMEDY

Reflexology has been shown to be very effective in reducing the severity of chronic back pain.[12] I've worked with many clients who complained about acute and chronic back pain for years and after just a few reflexology sessions could not believe the improvement and relief they felt. The great thing about reflexology is that it offers an effective way to affect areas of your spine that you could never reach yourself. By stimulating the corresponding reflex areas on your feet, you can soothe your entire spine and relax your body.

1. Take one foot in your hands and place your thumbs on the inside arch of the foot. Alternating thumbs, press your thumbs along the inner edge of your foot, concentrating on the areas that feel most tender on the foot; these areas correspond to the areas of your back that need it the most:

    > For lower-back pain, focus on the area along the inner sole between the heel and the middle of the foot.

    > For middle-back pain, focus on the middle section of the inner edge.

    > For upper-back problems, including neck pain, work the area along the inner edge of the foot from the base of the big toe to the middle of the foot.

2. To stimulate the entire back, begin at the heel and thumb-walk up the inner edge of the foot all the way to the base of the big toe (thumb-walking is alternately rubbing one thumb, then the other, as you slowly move your thumbs up the foot). Do this several times, spending extra time on any area that feels tender or "grainy." These areas may be congested, and they need it the most.

3. Repeat on the other foot.

4. *Alternate method:* If the inner soles of your feet are sensitive and tender to the touch, try rolling the arch of each foot on a tennis ball. The pressure of the tennis ball can stimulate the reflex areas to the spine just as well as your fingers. By leaning some of your body weight on the ball, you can control the pressure and help the ball sink deeper into your foot. This is a very relaxing yet invigorating way to start the day.

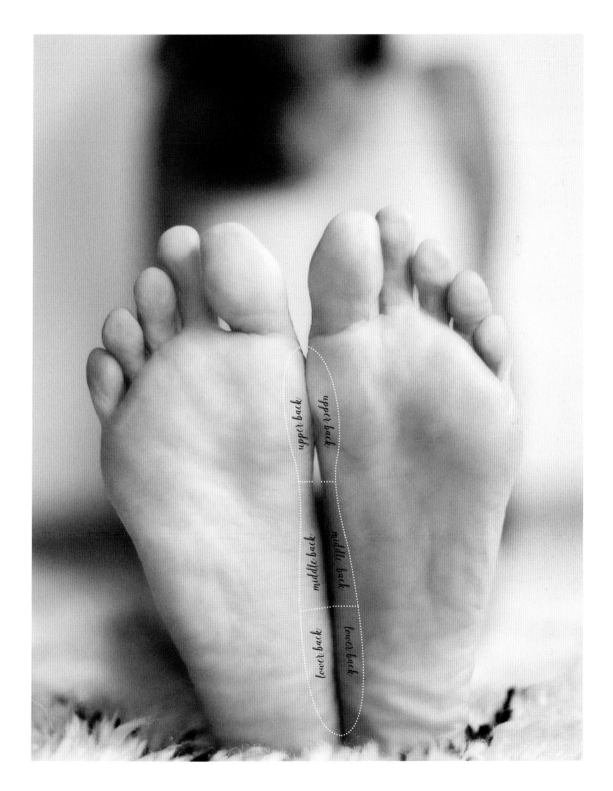

upper back

upper back

middle back

middle back

lower back

lower back

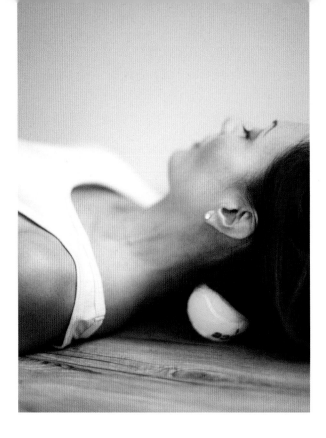

BACK-PAIN CRANIAL-SACRAL REMEDY

1. Lie on the floor and place a tennis ball under your back on either side of the spine at the bony ridge at the base of the spine (the sacrum). Either extend your legs straight out or keep your feet on the floor, knees bent, whichever feels most comfortable. Position yourself so that you feel a gentle pull in your lower back. Close your eyes, take a few deep breaths, and allow your body to let go.

2. Slowly rock back and forth on the balls. This provides a gentle mobilization to your spine and improves the flow of spinal fluid between your sacrum and head. This releases tension in the lower back, nourishes the brain, and relaxes the central nervous system. Reposition the balls slightly higher up your back and relax. Repeat this all the way up to your neck. When you reach your neck, hold still in this position for 10 to 15 seconds to allow the ball to sink deeper into the base of your neck, just below your skull.

NOTE: *You can also put the two tennis balls in a sock and tie the sock, close to the balls. Place the balls on either side of your spine as before. The sock prevents the balls from rolling out from under you.*

Fatigue and Low-Energy Remedies: Boost Your Energy Instantly

Everyone goes through periods in life when they feel exhausted, lethargic, sleepy, and unmotivated. Believe me, I've had my fair share. This feeling of low energy, also known as fatigue, can be caused by many things—overwork, trauma, general stress—and it usually goes away after some relaxation and a good night's sleep or two. However, the NIH says that approximately one in every five Americans claims to have fatigue that is severe enough to interfere with daily normal life. Experts say that one in ten people suffer from persistent tiredness (also known as TATT, "tired all the time" syndrome), and women are more likely to be affected than men.[13] There's also chronic fatigue syndrome, which affects approximately one million people in the United States, according to estimates from the CDC.[14]

Whether you suffer from occasional fatigue that leaves you feeling drained and unable to concentrate or fatigue has become a long-term problem that affects your quality of life and day-to-day activities, these remedies can help give you an energy boost. The acupressure remedy stimulates energy points on your belly, back, and shins. The reflexology remedy stimulates your adrenals, thyroid, and solar plexus. And the lymphatic massage remedy wakes up your lymphatic system to perk you up.

ANTI-FATIGUE ACUPRESSURE REMEDY

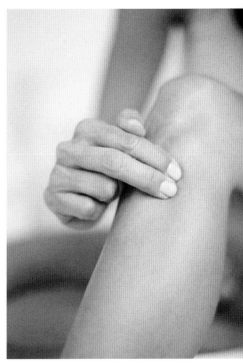

Three Mile Point

I. *"Three Mile" point:* Measure 3 finger-widths below your kneecap, and press your index and middle fingers in the area just 1 finger-width to the outer edge of your shinbone. Press firmly for 10 seconds, then make small circles in one direction, and then the other for another 10 to 20 seconds each. This helps boost your energy.

2. *"Sea of Vitality" point:* Reach your hands around to your middle back and bring your thumbs to your spine. Find your last rib (which is about ½ to 1 inch above the waist-line), move your thumbs slightly below the last rib, and about 2 finger-widths away from the spine. Press firmly for 10 seconds, release, and move your thumbs two more finger-widths away from the spine. Press there for 10 seconds and release. Alternate firm pressure on these four points. This can relieve fatigue and perk you up.

ANTI-FATIGUE REFLEXOLOGY REMEDY

....

1. *Thyroid reflex point:* Take your foot in one hand and bend your big toe back slightly. You'll notice that just under the ball of your foot there's a slight bulge. Press all along this bulge for 10 to 20 seconds to stimulate the reflex area to your thyroid and give yourself an energy boost. Repeat on the other foot.

2. *Solar plexus reflex point:* With your thumbs, press firmly in the center of the sole of your foot for 10 seconds. Make small circles in one direction and then the other for 20 seconds each. This is the reflex area to the solar plexus, the nerve center of your body, and stimulating it can increase your energy. Repeat on the other foot.

3. *Adrenals reflex point:* Move your thumbs just above the solar plexus point and you'll find the reflex area to the adrenals. Again, press and hold for 10 seconds, then make small circles in one direction and then the other for 20 seconds each. Stress causes the adrenals to release adrenaline and cortisol, and if you're always stressed, your adrenals are working overtime. Stimulating this area on both feet can open the energy channels to the adrenals and revive your energy.

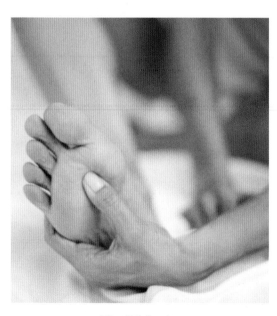

Thyroid Reflex Area

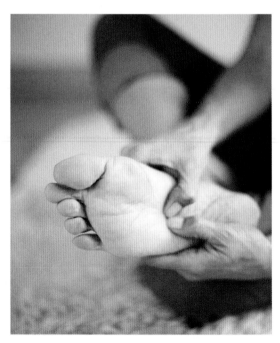

Solar Plexus Reflex Area

ANTI-FATIGUE LYMPHATIC MASSAGE REMEDY

I. Roll up your sleeves. Using your fingernails, lightly and quickly brush your other hand and arm, moving up toward your shoulder. (Do *not* brush downward.) It's almost as if you were brushing lint off a sweater, but with the tips of your fingernails. You shouldn't scratch yourself, but press firmly enough so you feel your skin is stimulated. Do this for a minute or so and then switch arms.

2. Next, do the same brushing motion all over your chest, moving down toward your heart. (Do *not* brush upward.) This stimulates your lymphatic system and helps wake you up. I like to do this in this morning to wake up and later when the afternoon slump begins.

ENERGY-BOOSTING AROMATHERAPY FOR FATIGUE

3 drops grapefruit oil
2 drops ginger oil
1 drop peppermint oil
2 ounces unscented natural oil

To further boost your energy, mix these stimulating essential oils together and rub a few drops between your fingertips. Inhale the scent, then follow the directions for each remedy. The invigorating scent will revitalize you instantly.

Headache Remedies: Soothe & Prevent Headaches!

Every year forty-five million people suffer from chronic headaches (twenty-eight million from migraines) and more than ten million people visit a doctor or the ER because of a headache.[15] Whether caused by stress, muscle tension, eyestrain, sinuses, hormones, or your significant other (just kidding . . . sort of), a headache can stop you in your tracks if you're not careful. As someone who used to suffer from regular migraines, I can tell you that there are effective, drug-free touch-therapy remedies that can help headaches. Studies now prove that massage therapy, especially stimulation of active trigger points, is helpful in relieving frequent chronic tension headaches. According to researchers leading one study: "The muscle-specific massage therapy technique used in this study has the potential to be a functional, non-pharmacological intervention for reducing the incidence of chronic tension headache."[16]

These touch-therapy remedies are very effective in relieving and preventing many headache symptoms, including pain, nausea, and pressure. People always ask me if the remedies will take their headache away immediately. Although everyone is different, the relaxation that touch therapy brings has a way of decreasing pain very quickly and successfully. I've found that if I can identify the signs of a headache coming on before it actually hits (i.e., pressure near my temples, zigzag lines in my peripheral vision, blurred vision—it's different for everyone), then I can use one of the remedies to ward off a full-blown headache. I've used the following remedies almost daily for many years, and I can honestly say that my headaches, which used to be quite debilitating, are a thing of the past. Seriously, I can't remember the last time I had one! Try using these trigger-point, reflexology, and acupressure remedies for soothing relief, so you can think clearly again.

HEADACHE TRIGGER-POINT REMEDY

1. Reach behind your head and place your thumbs on either side of the spine, just under the bony ridge (called the occipital ridge) at the base of your skull. Press firmly as you slowly tilt your head forward and back. As you lean your head back, you'll feel your thumbs moving deeper. Do this several times, then move your thumbs out toward your ears about ½ inch and repeat dropping your head forward and backward. Keep the pressure firm. Do this until you reach the edge of your skull close to your ears. Trigger points in this suboccipital muscle group are the most common cause of tension headaches.

2. Next, place your index and middle fingers at the base of your skull, on either side of your neck, just below your ears, which is the top of the sternocleidomastoid (SCM) muscle, which runs down the sides of your neck. Apply firm pressure for 10 seconds then move your fingers down the muscle about ½ inch. Again, apply pressure for 10 seconds and repeat all the way down the muscle until you reach the collarbone. Then repeat the same pressure, hold, release back up the SCM. The SCM has seven trigger points, making it one of the most highly concentrated trigger-point areas in the body.

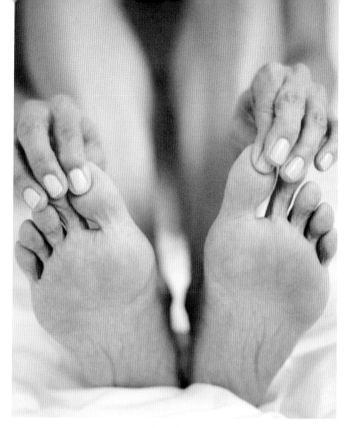

Brain Reflex Area

HEADACHE REFLEXOLOGY REMEDY

1. *Brain reflex point:* This reflex point is located on the big toe of both feet, in the fleshy part behind the toenail. Pinch both big toes with your index fingers on the pads of the toes and your thumbs on the nails for 10 seconds. Release and repeat. You can also make small circles with your thumb in the flesh of the big toe. For more pressure, I recommend using plastic clips (like "chip clips" or even clothespins), which you can snap onto your big toes. Pressing here will release congested energy and ease your aching head.

2. *Eye reflex point:* This reflex point is located at the area between the base of the second and third toes on both feet. Apply pressure with your thumbs for 10 seconds, release, and then make small circles with your thumbs. This can relieve headaches due to eyestrain.

3. *Neck reflex point:* This reflex point is located at the base of the big toe on both feet. Apply pressure for 10 seconds and then make small circles with your thumbs. This increases circulation to the neck and relieves headaches.

HEADACHE ACUPRESSURE REMEDY

....

1. *"Union Valley" points:* Apply pressure to the web between your thumb and index finger (pinching it between your other thumb and index finger) for 10 seconds, then make small circles with your thumb in one direction, then the other for another 10 seconds. I like to do this two ways: first with my thumb on the top of my hand and my index finger on the palm side, and then reversed, with my thumb on the palm side and index finger on top. Repeat on the other hand. Firm pressure on this area releases tension from head and neck.

2. *"Drilling Bamboo" points:* With your index fingers, apply pressure to the indentations on either side of the area where the bridge of the nose meets the ridge of the eyebrows for 10 seconds. Release and repeat. This helps to relieve headaches caused by eyestrain and sinus pain.

3. *"Gates of Consciousness" points:* Bring your index and middle fingers to the back of your head and place them underneath the base of the skull, in the hollows on both sides of the neck, between the two vertical neck muscles. Press upward on both sides for 10 seconds, release, and repeat. You can apply fairly strong pressure.

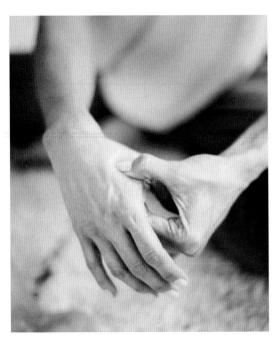

Union Valley

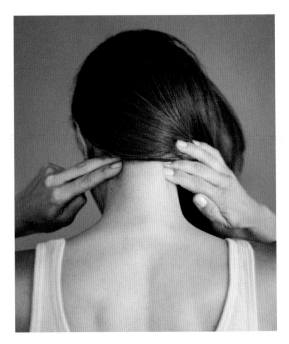

Gates of Consciousness

AROMATHERAPY FOR HEADACHES
....

4 drops spearmint oil
8 drops lavender oil
2 drops eucalyptus oil
2 ounces unscented natural oil

Before doing the headache remedies, I suggest rubbing a few drops of this powerful blend between your fingertips and inhaling the scent for a minute. As you do the remedies, the lingering scent on your fingertips will soothe your nerves. Be careful not to get too close to your eyes, as they may be sensitive to these essential oils.

Heart Problem Remedies: Nurture a Happy & Healthy Heart

It's obvious: stress is just not good for your heart. Period. It not only raises your blood pressure and produces damaging stress hormones, but studies also link it to changes in the way blood clots, which makes a heart attack more likely.[17] If you're chronically stressed and do nothing about it, you're more likely to have heart disease, high blood pressure, chest pain, or irregular heartbeats.[18] In our high-stress world about eighty million Americans have heart disease or high blood pressure, and over six hundred thousand people die of heart disease in the United States every year—that's one in every four deaths! Heart disease is the leading cause of death for both men and women, and its prevalence increases with age.[19] So it makes sense that anything that reduces stress, including all touch therapy, is beneficial for your heart.

In traditional Chinese medicine, emotions are considered the major internal causes of disease, and certain organs are related to particular emotional activities. The heart is said to be the seat of the soul. It's the organ in our body that's related to the feeling of joy, and its well-being is essential to our emotional balance, sexuality, and overall physical health. Therefore, it's extremely important to de-stress your life as much as possible, so that this muscle stays strong. After all, it's the hardest-working muscle in your body, pumping 2 ounces of blood at every heartbeat, or at least 2,500 gallons daily. Take care of it with these Swedish massage, reflexology, and therapeutic-touch remedies.

If you have a heart condition, you should always talk to your doctor before beginning a personal massage program.

HEART SWEDISH MASSAGE REMEDY

1. You will have to either undress or wear shorts, so that you can reach your thighs. Warm some oil or lotion in your hands and either sit comfortably in a chair or sit up in bed. (Place a towel under yourself if you're using oil.) Place both hands on the top of one ankle and stroke upward from the ankle, wrapping your hands around the back of your leg and stroking up your calf. Apply medium-firm pressure on the calf muscle. When you reach the knee, wrap your hands to the front of your shin and massage down to the ankle with very light pressure. Repeat this stroke several times. This encourages blood flow up the leg toward the heart.

2. Next, repeat stroking just from your knee to your upper thigh, using both hands to glide up the back of your leg (encouraging blood flow in the hamstrings to move in the direction of the heart) and then up the top of your leg (encouraging blood flow in the quadriceps to flow toward the heart.) As you glide your hands from the upper thigh back to knee, lighten your pressure. Repeat on the other leg. By massaging the leg muscles, you can improve your circulation and stimulate blood flow from your lower body back toward your heart.

HEART REFLEXOLOGY REMEDY

1. Take your left foot in your hands and place your thumbs on the area below your fourth and pinkie toes, closer to the outer edge of the foot and about halfway between the bottom of your pinkie toe and the middle of your foot.

2. Press your thumbs alternately using firm but gentle pressure in this area. Then, use your thumbs to make small circles in one direction and then the other for 10 to 20 seconds each way.

3. Next, alternate your thumbs as they stroke outward and upward, at a 45-degree angle, forming a "V," for another 20 seconds. Stimulate this reflex area to improve blood circulation and strengthen your heart.

NOTE: *Do not repeat on the other foot as the heart reflex is only on the left foot. On your right foot, this area corresponds to the liver reflex.*

HEART THERAPEUTIC-TOUCH REMEDY

Studies show that therapeutic touch has a positive effect on the vital signs of patients before coronary-artery bypass graft surgery. Researchers stated: "[Therapeutic touch] can be used as a simple, cheap and applicable technique in all health-care centers to help these patients."[20]

1. Lie comfortably on your back (clothes on or off—it's up to you). Rub the palms of your hands together to create warmth, then place them on your chest in any position that is comfortable for you. Take a deep breath in and slowly breathe out. Close your eyes and focus your attention on the warm energy surrounding your chest. Continue to take slow, deep inhalations and exhalations. If you're not used to meditation, this may be difficult, but try to imagine your body letting go of all tension with every exhale.

2. Remain in this position for 10 minutes. I like to set a timer so that I'm not thinking about the time. After 10 minutes I usually feel that my heart is beating slower, my breathing is deeper and longer, and my mind is clearer. This stress reliever is so good for the health of your heart.

Immunity Remedies: Don't Let Stress Knock You Down

Whenever I'm really stressed-out, I get sick. However, the strange thing is that it usually doesn't hit me while the stressful situation is happening, but rather a few weeks later, when I can relax (typically when I'm on vacation, which is great). I'm convinced that my body won't let me get sick because "I have to keep it together," until I don't have to keep it together anymore and I fall apart. That's just my theory.

However, a more scientific explanation comes from a recent study from Stanford University School of Medicine scientist Firdaus Dhabhar, who proved that short-term stress, such as that of the fight-or-flight response, could actually heighten, rather than suppress, your immune response. This study revealed that short-term stress stimulates immune activity, which is crucial for wound healing and preventing or fighting infection (which is maybe why I don't get sick), and both wounds and infections are common risks during chases, escapes, and combat.[21] However, the key word here is "short-term." In the long-term, chronic stress suppresses the immune system.

It's well known that stress, specifically the stress hormone cortisol, reduces your immune system's ability to fight off antigens, so you're more susceptible to infections. Stress may also have an indirect effect on the immune system, as stressed-out individuals may turn to unhealthy behaviors to cope with their stress, such as drinking, drugs, smoking, or overeating. Recent studies have shown that chronic inflammation, which is the immune system's response to injury or irritation, may be involved in everything from heart disease and diabetes to Alzheimer's disease and other forms of dementia.[22]

You've heard it a thousand times (probably even in this book): stress is bad for you. This touch-therapy remedy can help you reduce stress and stimulate your body's immune system, so you're better equipped to fight off disease and stay healthy.

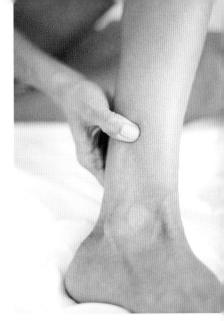

Three Yin Crossing

IMMUNITY ACUPRESSURE REMEDY

I. Using your thumb or index and middle fingers, press firmly on each of these following points for 10 seconds, then release, and make small circles in one direction and then the other for 10 seconds. Repeat several times on both feet.

"Three Mile" point is located about 3 finger-widths below the bottom of your kneecap, on the outside of your shinbone. You'll feel a slight depression and this point may be tender. This is one of the most powerful points for boosting immunity in the entire body, and I recommend stimulating this point on a daily basis. It increases energy, or *chi,* in the entire body, tones the blood, and calms the spirit.

"Three Yin Crossing" point is located about 4 finger-widths above the middle of your anklebone on the outside of your ankle. This is a powerful point for strengthening the spleen and stomach and boosting the immune system.

"Elegant Mansion" points are the depressions directly below the bottom of your collarbone (where the bones protrude). These two powerful points strengthen the immune system as well as help the respiratory system.

AROMATHERAPY TO STRENGTHEN
THE IMMUNE SYSTEM

....

6 drops lavender oil
6 drops bergamot oil
3 drops lemon oil
3 drops tea tree oil
2 ounces unscented natural oil

Before doing the immunity remedies, I suggest rubbing a few drops of this powerful blend between your fingertips and inhaling the scent for a minute. The remaining oil on your fingertips will be massaged into the acupressure points as you do the remedies.

Insomnia and Sleeping Remedies: Stop Counting Sheep!

There's nothing worse than lying in bed and watching the digits change on the clock as you count the dwindling hours until you have to get up. Stress is interfering with our sleep, and it's a real problem that affects both men and women (women are almost twice as likely to suffer from insomnia).[23] According to the NIH, 40 percent of the general population have problems falling asleep and 10 percent have symptoms of daytime functional impairment caused by insomnia, which means millions of people are going through their days drowsy and unfocused.

No matter your age or gender, a lack of sleep can throw your system off balance and lead to more serious problems including heart disease, high blood pressure, diabetes, depression, decreased libido, and memory loss. Sleep is not a luxury but a basic need, and touch can help!

Studies at the Touch Research Institute show that massage increases delta waves, those linked with deep sleep.[24] That's why it's so easy to fall asleep during a massage. It's too bad we can't all be massaged to sleep every night by a personal massage therapist. Yet, with these touch remedies, now you can! In addition, studies indicate acupressure is effective in relieving insomnia and significantly reducing the frequency of night awakenings.[25]

TOUCH THERAPY REDUCES STRESS AND STIMULATES YOUR BODY'S IMMUNE SYSTEM.

Try these touch remedies to help you turn off stress, so you can fall asleep and stay asleep. They're a drug-free alternative to endlessly counting sheep.

INSOMNIA AND SLEEP ACUPRESSURE REMEDY

I. Apply firm pressure with your thumbs to each of these two acupressure points, one at a time, for 10 seconds; then make small circles with your thumbs for another 10 seconds.

> *"Joyful Sleep" (or "Illuminated Sea") point* is located on the inside of the ankle where there is a slight indentation just below the anklebone.

> *"Calm Sleep" point* is located on the outside of the ankle just below your anklebone.

2. Then simultaneously press on these acupressure points, placing your thumb on one side and your index and middle fingers on the other side of your ankle and squeezing for 10 seconds. Stimulating these points before you go to bed can help relax your body, sedate your energy, and counter-act insomnia.

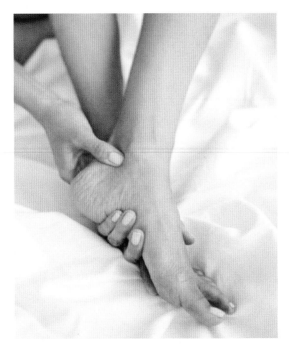

Joyful Sleep

AROMATHERAPY FOR INSOMNIA

....

2 drops bergamot oil
2 drops lavender oil
2 drops patchouli oil
2 drops ylang ylang oil
2 ounces unscented natural oil

This is my favorite aromatherapy blend for sleep. However, you may also consider mixing just a few drops of jasmine oil into unscented oil. Research from a recent study at Wheeling Jesuit University in West Virginia found that people who were exposed to the scent of jasmine had better-quality sleep than those who slept in a lavender-scented or odor-free room.[26]

INSOMNIA CRANIAL-SACRAL REMEDY

....

I. Lie flat on your back on the floor with knees bent and feet on the floor. Place a tennis ball under the back of your neck, as close as possible to the base of your skull (called the occipital ridge). There's an indentation you will feel where the ball fits perfectly. Allow the weight of your head and neck to sink into the ball for a minute or two.

2. Lift the tops of your feet, shift your weight onto your heels, and slowly roll your body forward and backward, so the ball gently massages the neck area and gives a nice stretch to the membranes underneath. This is a very subtle movement. Try not to lift your head, as the idea is to allow the weight of your head to press the tennis ball against the back of your neck. Using your legs to shift your body forward and back, the ball should roll only 1 or 2 inches at most. This encourages the flow of cerebrospinal fluid throughout the cranial-sacral system (your spine to your brain) and moves the autonomic nervous system from a highly aroused sympathetic-dominant state to a relaxed parasympathetic-dominant state. In other words, it calms your body down so you can sleep.

3. When you feel sufficiently relaxed, crawl into bed.

Remedies for Weight Issues: Gaining or Losing

Stress and weight issues go hand in hand. Whether you're a "gainer" or a "loser," touch therapy, specifically acupressure and reflexology, can help you manage your weight. When you're stressed, there's no question that your endocrine system is under fire, causing you to do things that you probably shouldn't do (like eating a second piece of cake). In a nutshell, when you're stressed, your adrenal glands, which govern your "stress response," release a cascade of hormones, including adrenaline, cortisol, and corticotropin-releasing hormone (CRH), into your body. In the short term, the adrenaline helps you feel less hungry as blood flows away from your organs and goes to your heart and large muscles to prepare for "fight or flight." However, in the longer term, when the adrenal glands are overworked and the effects of the adrenaline wear off, cortisol (the stress hormone) signals your body to prepare for disaster by storing fat and calories. This is when you crave food, lose precious energy, and gain weight.[27]

Whether you want to lose weight or gain weight, a key element in both processes is your metabolism. Metabolism, which takes place in your muscles and organs, is essentially your body's process of converting food into energy. It's the speed at which your body's motor is running—to lose weight, you must try to increase your metabolism, and to gain weight, you must slow your metabolism. For centuries, the Chinese and Japanese have successfully used these reflexology and acupressure techniques to help regulate metabolism, control appetite, and manage weight issues. I first learned of them over thirty years ago when the Japanese exchange student who was living with my family showed me her "tricks" to staying slim. I'm happy to pass them on to you!

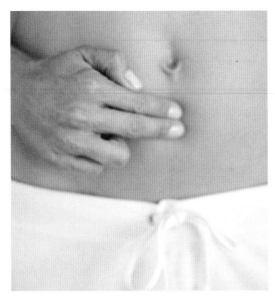
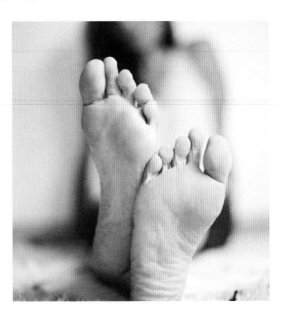

Sea of Energy

WEIGHT ACUPRESSURE REMEDY

....

I. Apply pressure for 30 seconds with your thumb or index and middle
fingers to the following points. Then make small circles in one direction
and then the other for another 1 to 2 minutes. Do this several times each
day for best results.

> The *"Sea of Energy" point* is located 3 finger-widths below your belly
> button. This powerful point enhances the function of the digestive
> system, reduces constipation, and energizes your metabolism.

> *"Abdominal Sorrow" points* are located above the stomach and just below
> your rib cage. If you were to follow a vertical line down each nipple,
> these two points are about ½ inch toward the midline of the body.
> Stimulating these points can help control your appetite, reduce indi-
> gestion, and relieve ulcers.

> *"Appetite Control" points* are located just in front of your ear. To find
> them, place your middle and index fingers against your jaw, right
> in front of your ears, on either side of your face, and open and close
> your mouth. These pressure points are exactly where there is the most
> movement; they help to control appetite.

WEIGHT REFLEXOLOGY REMEDY

....

I. *Thyroid reflex area:* This area is located on the soles of both feet about 1
inch from the inside of the inner edge of the foot and about 1 inch below
the crease between your big toe and second toe. Press this area and make
small circles for 15 seconds. Stimulate this area to boost your metabolism.

2. *Pineal reflex area:* This reflex area is located at the base of the big toe on
both feet, toward the inner edge. Make small circles here for 15 seconds,
release, and repeat. Stimulate this area to suppress an overactive appetite.

3. *Kidney, liver, colon, and small intestine reflex areas:* These reflex areas are located
on the soles of both feet, in the middle of the foot. The best way to reach
all of these areas is to roll your foot over a tennis ball several times. It's best
to do this barefoot, so there is some traction. Stand up so that you can apply
pressure as you roll the ball. This helps with detoxification and elimination.

Take care of your body. It's the only place you have to live.
—JIM ROHN

WE LEAVE TRACES OF OURSELVES WHEREVER WE GO,

ON WHATEVER WE TOUCH.

—LEWIS THOMAS

CHAPTER FOUR

Women's Remedies

Nurture the Nurturers

In most families today, women are the primary caretakers—the loving, accommodating nurturers responsible for making sure everyone is healthy and happy. Sounds familiar, right? Even though traditional roles within the family are slowly evolving and many men are stay-at-home dads, women are still the ones who carry and breast-feed the baby and often give up careers to stay home and care for the children. Women also provide the majority of informal care to spouses, parents, in-laws, friends, and neighbors, acting simultaneously as a hands-on caregiver, health manager, companion, and advocate. With this long list of people to care for, we frequently fail to care for ourselves.

The touch remedies in this chapter are my most valuable massage techniques to help women take care of themselves while taking care of others. I've used each and every one of these remedies hundreds of times, and they definitely come in handy on those occasions when I feel as though I'm falling apart and need a time-out.

On top of the stresses of caring for others, many of us are deprived of the nonsexual, compassionate, loving touch that everyone so desperately needs, even with kids literally hanging on us all day long. This, in turn, can lead to even more stress.[1] When we're stressed to the point of burnout, the brain's fear center is activated and we lose emotional control. According to Joan Borysenko, a Harvard-trained scientist and psychologist: "Burnout is a disorder of hope. It sucks the life out of competent, hard-working people. You lose motivation and vitality."[2] I say that it's about time for women to start noticing the warning signs and take swift action to reduce stress before it gets to this point!

No matter what stage of life you're at or how good you think you are at multitasking, every woman needs and deserves attention, support, and a little "me time" to refuel her body, mind, and spirit. Women of all ages *need* to understand that it's okay to take a break and nurture themselves. Instead of feeling guilty, women must give themselves permission to relax, make time for themselves, and learn how to provide their own stress relief on a daily basis.

My touch remedies are valuable tools women can use to take control of their health and make fundamental changes to their lifestyle. As women age, their bodies change, and more demands are put on them, different problems may arise that can be physically and mentally damaging. This chapter includes touch-therapy remedies that address the specific problems in each stage of a woman's life. They're easy and effective and don't take more than a few minutes of your time.

In "Pregnancy," you'll find self-massage and partner massage techniques for common problems that arise during those challenging nine months. "Moms" contains quick touch remedies to help boost energy, clear up "mommy brain," and help you sleep. In "Aging Beautifully," there are remedies women of any age can use to help them look and feel better, and "Menopause and PMS Management" has touch remedies to help with mood swings, hot flashes and night sweats, and bone-density loss.

As a mother of three boys, I know what it's like to experience burnout and, believe me, I fight it every day. Minibreaks of just 5 minutes or less during which I can relieve some stress definitely make a big difference in my state of mind as the day unfolds. My touch remedies are part of my own arsenal of self-care stress relievers, and I'm thrilled to share them with you.

Pregnancy: Nine Months of Calm

A grand adventure is about to begin.
—WINNIE THE POOH

Ask any woman who has given birth and she'll tell you that the nine-plus months of pregnancy were some of the most exciting and rewarding but also physically and emotionally challenging and stressful months of her life. With three pregnancies under my belt, I can definitely vouch for that! In anticipation of a new baby, expectant mothers sometimes neglect their own well-being and focus mainly on "baby prep" and "family prep," if there are other siblings. I definitely did this when I was pregnant with baby number three! Yet all you pregnant women out there should know that nurturing yourself during this time is as important as caring for a newborn. A calm mom-to-be is essential to a healthy pregnancy, and no matter what's happening in your life, *it is possible* to find moments of relaxation and peace throughout the day. My safe and soothing touch remedies will help you find them.

During pregnancy, women suffer from all sorts of discomforts, including nausea, headaches, back pain, body aches, irritability, and depression. (I could go on, but I'll spare you the rest.) Traditional medicine offers few ways of alleviating these problems, but studies indicate that massage therapy during pregnancy can:

- Reduce stress and anxiety
- Relieve nausea
- Reduce headaches
- Relieve muscle aches, back pain, and joint pains
- Improve circulation
- Reduce swelling (edema)
- Improve sleep
- Decrease symptoms of depression
- Improve labor outcomes and newborn health[3]

Two studies by Tiffany Field, at the University of Miami's Touch Research Institute, showed just how beneficial massage can be during pregnancy. In one study, 26 pregnant women were assigned to a massage-therapy or a relaxation-therapy group for five weeks and received 20-minute sessions twice a week. Both groups reported feeling less anxious and less leg pain. However, only the massage-therapy group reported *reduced anxiety, improved mood, better sleep, and less back pain* by the end of the study. In addition, the

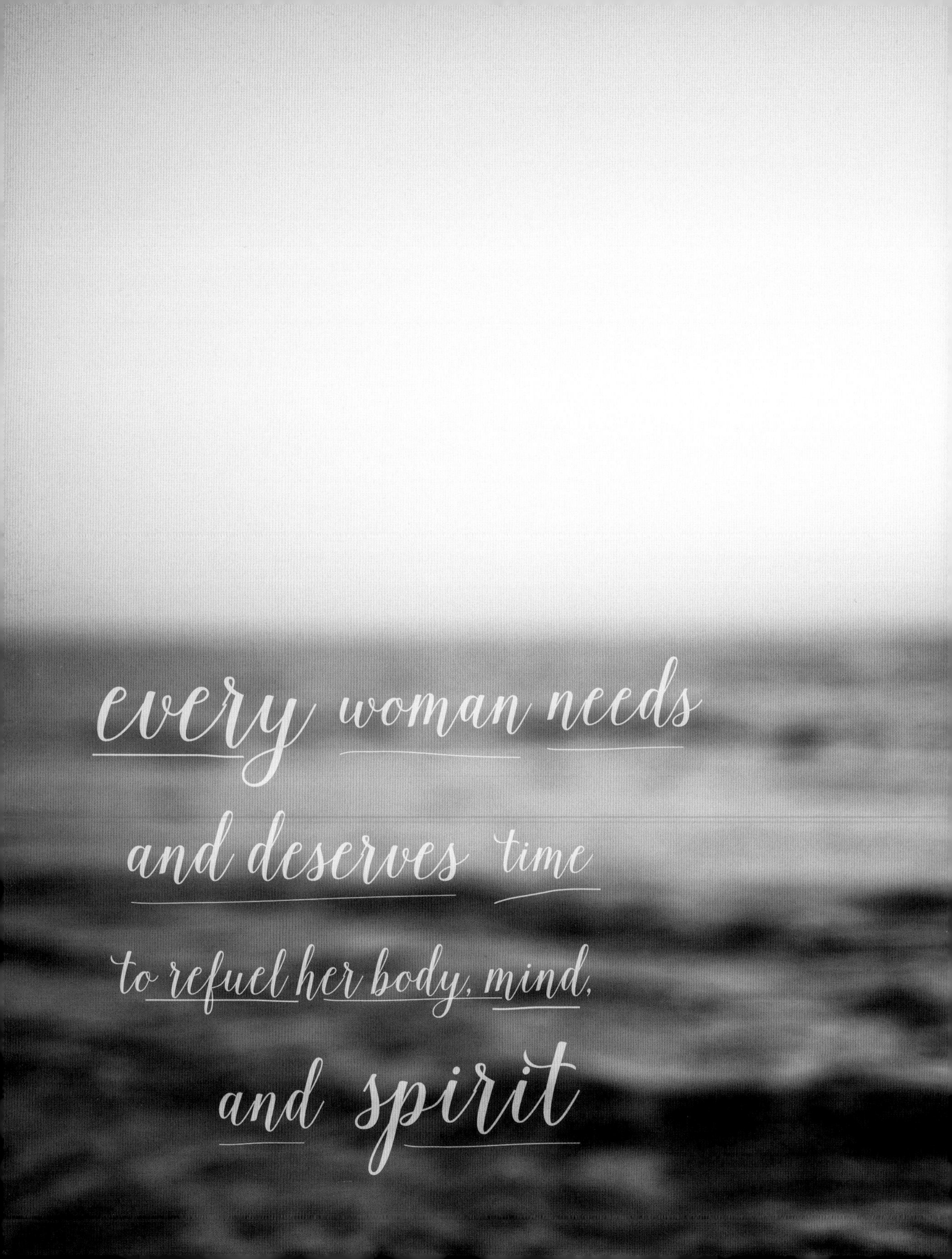

every woman needs

and deserves time

to refuel her body, mind,

and *spirit*

massage group had a decrease in urinary stress hormone levels (norepineph-rine) and fewer complications during labor, and their infants had fewer post-natal complications (e.g., less prematurity).[4] Wow! If that's not a reason to use massage during pregnancy, I don't know what is. But there's more.

In another study researchers found that massage therapy reduced pain (as well as depression, anxiety, and anger) in pregnant women, alleviated prena-tal depression in both parents, and improved their relationships. The partners who massaged the pregnant women reported less depressed mood, anxiety, and anger. The study stated, "These data suggest that not only mood states but also relationships improve mutually when depressed pregnant women are massaged by their partners."[5]

There are several different massage techniques (both self and partner) that can help pregnant women. By learning these simple techniques, moms-to-be can soothe their aches and pains and better cope with the changes of preg-nancy. In addition, pregnancy massage can bring much-needed touch to a mom-to-be at a time when her partner may be afraid to touch her for fear of hurting her or the baby. During this period, when both partners need a way to connect, touch can work wonders. Pregnancy massage also allows partners to feel helpful at a time when they really have no idea what to do.

The following touch remedies, treating nausea, swollen feet and ankles, headache, back pain, and stress relief, can help an expecting mom take charge of her pregnancy and feel more in control physically and emotionally. They're 100 percent safe and extremely effective. I used all of them throughout my three pregnancies, and I've used them on many expecting women. If you're expecting or know someone who is, I hope you'll take advantage of these pregnancy touch remedies and use them as much as necessary. And for those of you moms-to-be out there who may be experiencing discomfort or stress, remember, *this too shall pass!*

Pregnancy Precautions

1. As with any therapeutic approach to pregnancy health, women should discuss massage with their prenatal care provider.
2. The main *areas that you should avoid* during pregnancy are the reflex areas that are directly connected to the uterus and ovaries. These areas are located on the inside and outside of both feet, in the hollow areas just under the anklebones. Pressing here is a direct channel to these reproductive organs, so you do not want to mas-sage them during pregnancy. However, during labor these are areas you can massage to stimulate contractions and get labor started.

ANTI-NAUSEA ACUPRESSURE REMEDY

Nausea (or "morning sickness") is very common during pregnancy. During the first trimester about 25 percent of pregnant women suffer from nausea and 50 percent suffer from both nausea and vomiting. Normally, it all goes away by week fourteen, but some unlucky women suffer from it until delivery. No one knows for sure what causes it, but it's probably some combination of the many hormonal changes taking place in the body. In traditional Chinese medicine, morning sickness or nausea is seen as energy (*chi*) going in the wrong direction. Nausea and vomiting can definitely make you miserable and stressed-out during an already stressful time, so this self-acupressure technique can be a godsend for you (it was for me!).

I. *"Inner Gate" (P6) point:* Place your right thumb on your left wrist, about 2 finger-widths above the left wrist crease. Press deeply between the two tendons and hold for 20 to 30 seconds. If you can't see the tendons, bend

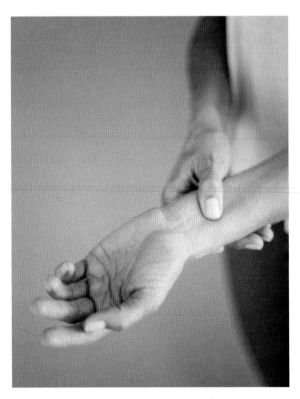

Inner Gate

your hand toward your elbow crease and form a claw with your fingers; this will bring the tendons up for you to see. Pressing on this acupressure point, which is connected to the stomach, can calm your mind and relieve nausea. Do this on both wrists. (This is the area that anti-nausea wristbands stimulate. And, yes, they do work!)

ANTI-NAUSEA REFLEXOLOGY REMEDY

Reflexology is also a very useful technique for soothing and healing yourself during pregnancy. If you can reach your feet (which I assume most people can do, that is until the baby belly takes over toward the end of the pregnancy!), then you can easily do self-reflexology.

I. *Stomach reflex area:* Press and hold your thumbs firmly on the inner edge of the foot, close to the middle of the foot, for 5 seconds, and then make small circles for about 5 seconds. Move your thumbs over about ½ inch and repeat the press to cover the entire reflex area to the stomach, which is like a half-moon that extends from about 2 inches below the big toe to about 2 inches above the heel, and reaches a third of the way to the center of the foot. Stimulating this area can help relieve nausea. Repeat on the other foot.

AROMATHERAPY FOR NAUSEA

3 drops of grapefruit oil
2 ounces unscented natural oil

Before doing the above touch remedies, rub a few drops of this aromatherapy blend between your fingertips. Take a few deep inhalations of the scent on your fingertips, and then proceed with the touch remedies.

You can also add a few drops of peppermint oil to water and keep it by your bed to smell when you wake up or whenever you feel nauseous. But do not put it on your skin, since peppermint oil is not recommended for topical use when pregnant.

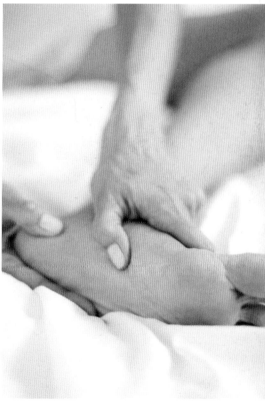

Stomach Reflex Area

NO-MORE-CANKLES LYMPHATIC MASSAGE REMEDY

Puffy ankles and feet are normal during pregnancy, especially during the third trimester when you're retaining water and the growing uterus is putting pressure on the pelvic veins, slowing the return of blood from the feet and legs to the heart. When this happens, excess fluid collects in the tissues (called edema) and causes swelling. It's normally worse at the end of the day and during the summer. This gentle lymphatic massage technique can improve circulation and help your body eliminate excess fluid. Studies show that manual lymph drainage (MLD) significantly reduced swelling of the legs of pregnant women and helped to reduce their limb size.[6] FYI, taking a break and elevating your feet can help too!

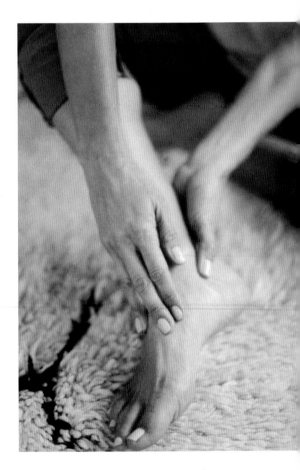

1. *On your own:* Sit with one ankle crossed over your leg, so that you can comfortably reach your foot. Warm some oil or lotion in your hands. Take your foot in the palms of your hands and vigorously rub the top and bottom of your foot and your ankle, using circular motions with firm pressure, for 30 seconds.

2. Move your hands to the ankle and continue the circular rubbing for 15 seconds. Then continue the circles up the leg to the knee.

3. Bring your hands back to the foot and alternate rubbing your thumb in a backward motion (toward you) starting on the sole of the foot, then the top of the foot, ankle, and lower leg. Try to cover every inch of skin with this thumb-rubbing technique.

4. With the tips of your fingers, apply firm pressure and brush upward from the toes to the knee several times. Do *not* go in the opposite direction. Always brush in the direction of the heart. Do this for 60 seconds. Switch feet.

5. Elevate both feet, lie back, and relax.

6. *With a partner:* Simply relax back with your legs stretched out in front of you. The most comfortable position is on a couch with your lower legs resting in your partner's lap. Partners should use the same vigorous circular motions, thumb rubbing, and fingertip brushing toward the knee. (Partners should remember to ask if the pressure is okay).

AROMATHERAPY FOR SWOLLEN FEET AND ANKLES

Soak your feet for 15 to 30 minutes in:

> 2 quarts of warm water
> 10 drops lavender oil
> 1 cup of Epsom salts

PREGNANCY HEADACHE REFLEXOLOGY REMEDY

Headaches during pregnancy are one of the most common discomforts and complaints. (I know, as I suffered with frequent migraines through all three pregnancies.) The surge of hormones combined with an increase in blood volume circulating throughout the body are typically the cause, along with lack of sleep, low blood sugar, dehydration, and . . . *stress.* Unfortunately, pregnancy is a time when women should avoid most headache medications. This is the perfect time to turn to natural remedies, such as these reflexology techniques, to soothe a headache without medication. You can do these on your own or have a partner do them for you.

1. *Brain reflex area:* Sit cross-legged and pinch the fleshy pad of each big toe with your thumb and index finger for 10 seconds. Release and repeat. Next, make small circles with your thumbs in the fleshy part of the big toes. Stimulating the reflex area to the brain can help release congested energy, soothe headaches, and send healing energy throughout the entire body.

2. *Neck reflex area:* Pinch both big toes between your thumbs and index fingers, roll them for 15 seconds, and make small circles rubbing along the base of the big toes for 15 seconds. Gently pinch the tips of each toe and pull out, so the fingers snap off. This stimulates the sinuses, which are sometimes congested during pregnancy. These are the main areas to focus on to relieve headaches.

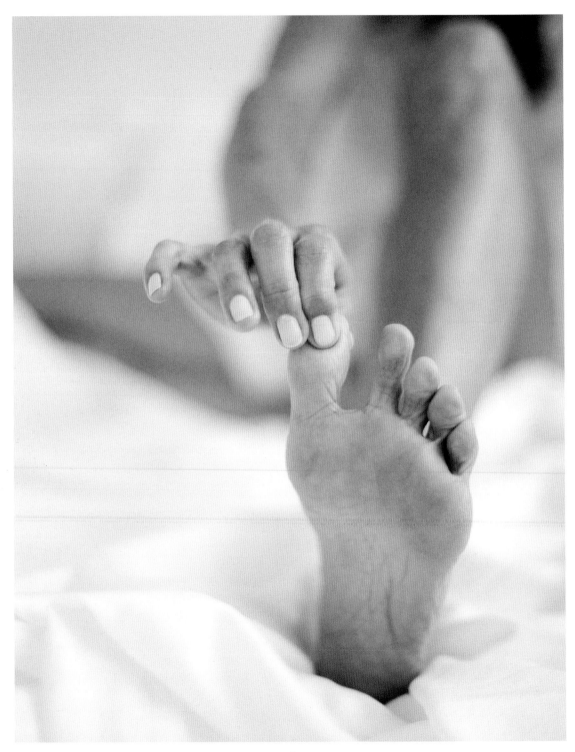

Brain Reflex Area

BACK-PAIN REFLEXOLOGY REMEDY

Backaches are very common during pregnancy, and they're particularly annoying since you can't take any medication to relieve the pain. Half of all pregnant women can expect some back pain, typically caused by poor posture, inappropriate lifting techniques, lack of exercise, the weight of the baby, and the softening of stretching ligaments to prepare for labor. As the baby grows, the hollow in your back may increase, and this can cause your back to ache. Also, due to the increased weight, the muscles in your back have to work harder to support your balance, which causes lower-back pain. Fortunately, there are several simple techniques you can use to ease the pain, one of which is reflexology. Here you will be working with the spinal reflex area.

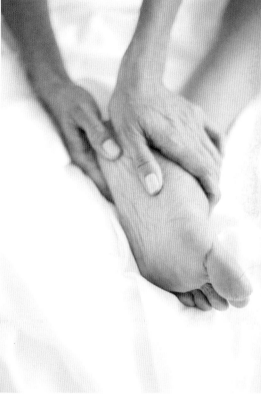

Back Reflex Area

1. Sit on a bed or chair so that your back is supported, but you can bend one leg and hold the foot in your hands. Place your thumbs on the inner edge of the foot, close to the heel, and press firmly, making small circles with your thumbs. Move your thumbs up about ½ inch and continue making small circles on the inner edge of the foot. Repeat all the way up to just below the big toe and then back down to the heel. Next, inch your thumb up and down the inner edge of the foot. This whole area along the inner edge of the foot is the reflex area to the spine. Pressing here can help relieve and even prevent back pain. Repeat on the other foot. (Your partner can also do this for you.)

2. Stand up and hold on to a chair for support. Place a tennis ball under one foot and gently roll the inner edge of your foot on the ball, allowing the weight of your body to add more or less pressure. This is a great way to stimulate the reflex area to the spine. Try to roll the ball to any other areas that may be tender or sensitive, gently relaxing your body weight onto the ball. This increases circulation to the entire body, especially areas of your back that are tight and achy.

BACK-PAIN SWEDISH MASSAGE REMEDY

With a partner, Swedish massage is the recommended prenatal massage method during pregnancy, because it addresses many common discomforts associated with the skeletal and circulatory changes a mom-to-be experiences during pregnancy. This technique can be done throughout pregnancy and during labor. It can help partners feel useful at a time when they don't know what to do. It helped me tremendously!

1. The mama-to-be should lie on her side, with a pillow in front of her belly, another between her legs, and a third under her head. Her top arm can rest on the pillow to bring her weight slightly forward. When she is comfortable, the partner can sit close to her lower back.

2. Partner, warm some oil in your hands and place the palms of both hands on her foot that lies on top. With medium pressure, slowly glide the palms of both hands up her leg to the top of her thigh and back down. Repeat several times to cover her entire leg. Spread your hands farther apart so your reach both the front and back of her leg. Repeat four or five times.

3. Next, move your hands up to her lower back and place your hands on either side of her spine. (If she's cold, cover her top leg with a towel or sheet.) Apply firm, gentle pressure as you massage up her back and around her shoulders. This position is a little awkward, and you may find it easier to place one hand on her shoulders for support and just massage up her back with your top hand. Either way, try to apply enough pressure to the muscles on the side of the spine (*never* on the spine directly) as you massage up to her neck and around her shoulders. This improves circulation and is deeply relaxing. Do this for as long as you want; then have her turn over and reposition the pillows, and massage her other side.

STRESS-RELIEF ACUPRESSURE REMEDY

Pregnancy brings out the neurotic worrier in all of us! No matter if this is your first or your fifth child, pregnancy can cause anxiety about everything from what you're eating and drinking and how you're feeling to whether the baby is healthy and how this baby will change your life and the lives of everyone around you. It happens to every mom-to-be, and the best thing you can do is find ways to manage your anxiety before it becomes all-consuming.

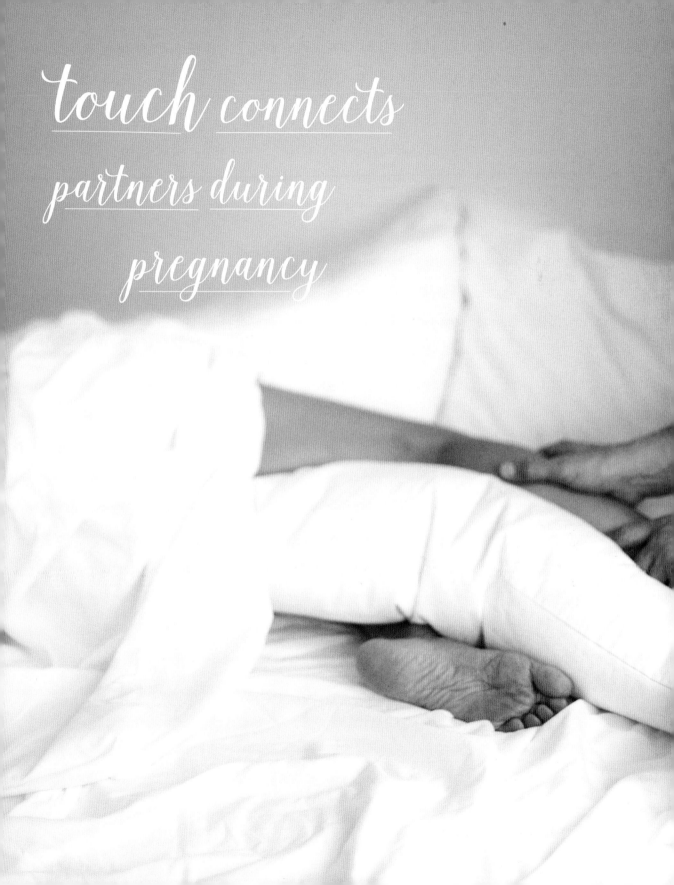

touch connects
partners during
pregnancy

Since studies show that a high level of chronic stress can boost the odds of preterm labor and of delivering a low-birth-weight baby, taking care of yourself and decreasing stress is essential to a healthy pregnancy. Touch remedies can not only relieve stress and anxiety, but also help with insomnia and fatigue. Use them during pregnancy and labor and for many years after.

A recent study showed that acupressure is an effective, noninvasive, and easily applicable technique to reduce labor pain. The study evaluated the effect of stimulating acupressure points on labor pain and duration during the first stage of labor.[7]

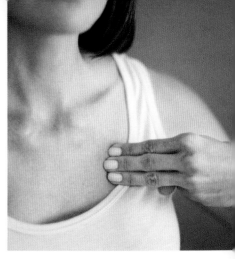

Letting Go

I. *"Letting Go" points:* Place the fingertips of your three middle fingers about 3 finger-widths below the collarbone on either side of your upper chest. Press firmly and make small circles with your fingers for 15 seconds.

2. Then, applying the same pressure, slowly drag your fingertips down your chest.

3. Repeat several times covering the area below the collarbone on both sides.

STRESS-RELIEF REFLEXOLOGY REMEDY

I. *On your own:* Bend one leg over the other and place your thumbs on the center of the sole of your foot. Press firmly for 10 seconds, then make small circles in one direction and then the other. Do this for several minutes; then switch feet and repeat on the other side. This stimulates the *reflex area to the solar plexus,* the "nerve center of the body." Pressing here can relax the entire body and bring instant stress relief.

2. *With a partner:* Partner, sit near the mama-to-be's feet and gently press one thumb into the center of each foot at the same time. Make small circles with your thumbs moving in one direction and then the other. Next, while you are pressing your thumb firmly into the center of the foot, use your other hand to slowly bend the foot over your thumb; which adds more pressure to the *solar plexus,* and then release it. Repeat several times.

A baby is something you carry inside you for nine months, in your arms
for three years, and in your heart till the day you die.

—MARY MASON

Solutions for Moms

Mothers are all slightly insane.
—J. D. SALINGER

I've said it before and I'll say it again: *Motherhood is freakin' stressful!* I know I'm not the only one who feels this way, since studies report that over 70 percent of moms in the United States say mothering is "incredibly stressful" and 96 percent feel that we're much more stressed than our own mothers were.[8] Whether you're a stay-at-home mom or a full-time working mom, a first-time mom or a mom of five, the juggling of family, work, finances, and life in general can leave you feeling exhausted, stressed, and out of control.

During motherhood, when you're pulled in a million different directions, it's easy to let stress invade your life. If you're a mom in your forties, which researchers describe as the new "rush hour of life"—when career and child-rearing peaks collide—stress can be unbearable. So in order to maintain a healthy body and preserve your sanity, it's essential that you *recognize* and *manage* stress before it becomes overwhelming and damaging to your health. In general, women are actually pretty good at recognizing stress, as studies show they're more likely than men to report physical and emotional symptoms of stress.[9] However, recognizing stress is one thing—dealing with it is another.

Unfortunately, most moms put everyone else's needs and desires before their own. They ignore their own stress and are left feeling frustrated, resentful, angry, and depressed. This all-too-common scenario has a "snowball effect," as stress not only hurts you, but your family too. Studies show that chronically stressed moms tend to be more insensitive toward kids. They also show that a mother's ability to manage stress is a strong predictor of the quality of her relationship with her children and how happy her children are.[10]

Since kids naturally imitate the behavior of their parents, how you manage stress is a model for the way they will handle it. Moms who handle stress in harmful ways (i.e., overeating, self-medicating with alcohol or drugs, smoking, compulsive shopping) may be able to alleviate their stress in the short run, but they can end up with significant health problems (and more stress) in the long run. Unhealthy behavior like this sets a poor example for children.

What I know for sure is this: in order for you to care for your family to the best of your ability, you *must* take care of yourself first! It's like when you're on an airplane and you're told to put the oxygen mask on yourself first and then on your kids. Remember: *you first,* kids second! To be the best mother you can be, you have to make yourself a priority and devote time to nurturing yourself each and every day. It's as much a gift to your kids and your family as it is to yourself. I know that when I spend a little part of my day nurturing myself, whether it's working out, reading a magazine, or giving myself a 5-minute foot massage, I'm a much more patient and loving mother and wife.

For that reason, I encourage you to take a break, nurture yourself every day, and manage your stress with a few of my touch remedies that will help you fight "mommy brain," boost your energy, and sleep better. Touch therapy can help you disconnect from the chaos that surrounds you and connect to the place of stillness and peace that lies within you. The following simple and quick remedies have helped me stay calm and balanced (most of the time) throughout my twelve years of motherhood with my three boys, and I hope they'll do the same for you!

"MOMMY BRAIN" CRANIAL-SACRAL REMEDY

"Mommy brain," the phenomenon of forgetfulness that often sets in even before you give birth, is a fact of life for most moms. If you have trouble remembering things that used to come easily and can't focus due to lack of sleep, stress, too many schedules, and the sheer chaos of kids, you probably have "mommy brain." This cranial-sacral remedy can help you relax and refocus your mind.

1. Behind your head, find the ridge at the base of your skull (the occipital ridge). Place the three middle fingers of each hand just under the ridge, on either side of your spine, and apply light pressure.

2. Tilt your head forward, still keeping the pressure, and then allow your head to slowly fall backward so that your fingertips gently massage under the ridge. This loosens up the area between the skull and the neck. Repeat four or more times.

3. Another way to open up this area is to put two tennis balls into a sock and tie the sock as close to the tennis balls as possible (so they can't move around). Lie on the floor and place the tennis balls just under the ridge below your skull (one ball on either side of your cervical spine). Let your head relax back, allowing the weight of the neck and head to be supported by the tennis balls, and extend your legs when you're comfortable. Relax in this position for 5 minutes. (You may fall asleep!)

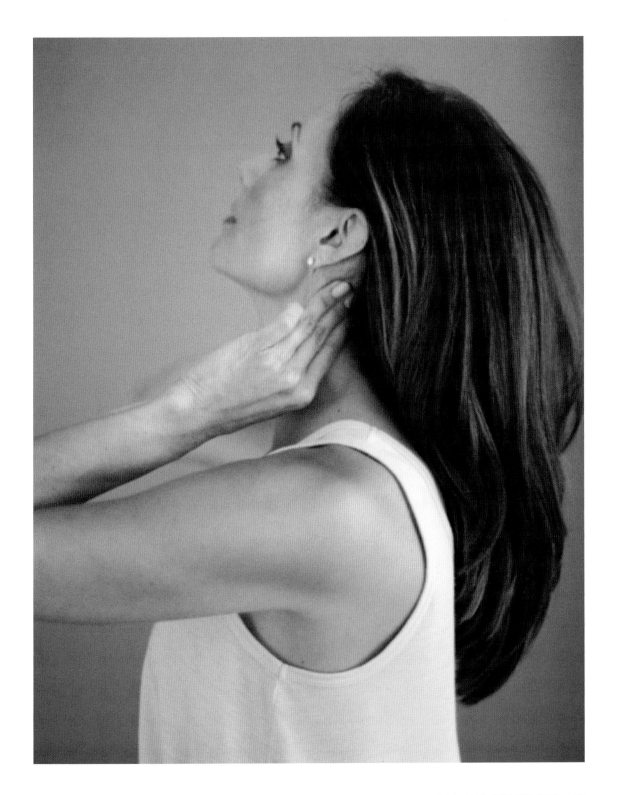

ENERGY-BOOSTING ACUPRESSURE REMEDY

Motherhood is one of the most physically and emotionally demanding jobs a woman will ever perform. The stress of changes in your body, caregiving, sleep deprivation, nursing, and ever changing family dynamics make this a particularly challenging period that can zap the energy right out of you. This acupressure technique can help rejuvenate your energy naturally, without sugar or caffeine, so you can make it through your day.

Studies show that acupressure can provide an effective natural energy boost. According to researcher Richard Harris: "[Acupressure] seems to stimulate the nerves that moderate attention and alertness." In this study, participants stimulated five acupressure points by tapping each point lightly with the fingertips for 2 or 3 minutes. The most effective point was the Si Shen Chong point, found right in the center of the top of the head.[11]

I. *"Si Shen Chong" point:* Using the fingertips of your three middle fingers of both hands, tap the very center of the top of your head lightly for 2 minutes. I usually set a timer and close my eyes while doing this.

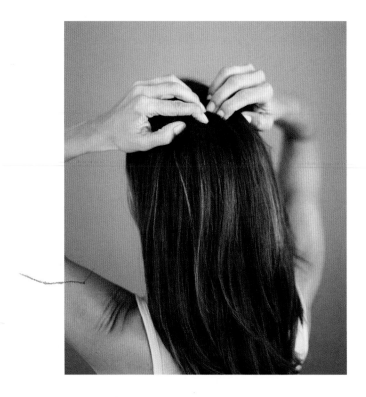

2. *"Middle of a Person" point:* This is another useful acupressure point to stimulate for an energy boost. It's located between your upper lip and nose, about one-third of the way down from the bottom of your nose. Apply firm pressure with the tip of one finger (or the tip of a fingernail for increased effectiveness) for 1 minute to increase your mental clarity and focus and revive your physical energy.

3. *Ear rub:* Your ears have acupressure points too! For more energy, firmly pinch each earlobe between your thumb and index finger and make small circles as you count to ten. Move your fingers slightly up the earlobe and repeat, continuing all the way up until you've covered the entire ear.

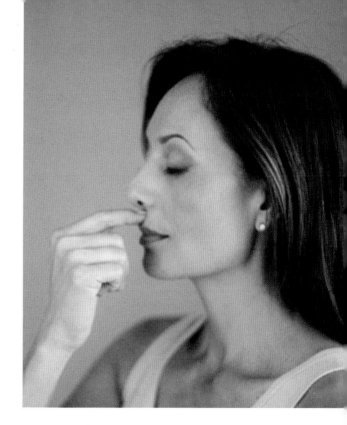

SLEEP BETTER ACUPRESSURE REMEDY

According to the National Sleep Foundation, over 58 percent of all Americans experience insomnia-like symptoms each week—and I'd bet a lot of them are moms! Whether it's due to insomnia, nighttime waking, or just not enough hours of rest, insufficient sleep really affects your ability to function, and it's been linked to all kinds of health problems, including obesity, diabetes, and heart disease. Studies have even compared the risks of driving drowsy with the risks of driving drunk—it's estimated to cause one hundred thousand auto accidents a year.[12] (I definitely remember feeling as though I shouldn't have been driving after several sleepless nights in a row nursing a newborn!)

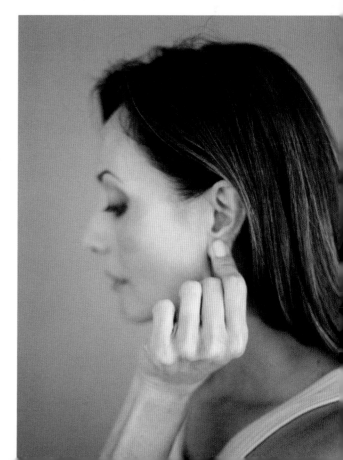

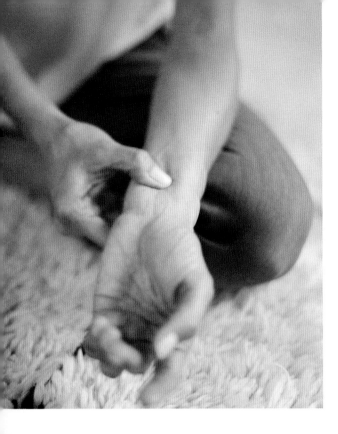

Women are already twice as likely as men to have difficulties falling and staying asleep, and during motherhood the changes in hormonal levels, needy kids, and stress only intensify this. It's time to take sleep as seriously for your health as diet and exercise and get some shut-eye!

1. *"Third Eye" point:* Between your eyebrows, there is a small depression on the level of your brows, above the nose. With your middle or index finger, apply gentle but firm pressure to that area for 1 minute. This can relieve anxiety, stress, and headaches, so you can sleep better.

2. *"Inner Gate" point:* On your left forearm, approximately 3 finger-widths above your wrist crease, place your right thumb between the two tendons. Apply moderate pressure with your right thumb, holding for 5 minutes and breathing deeply. Repeat on the other arm.

3. *"Peaceful Sleep" point:* Place your middle fingers behind your ears at the base of the skull, slightly above jaw level. You'll feel a slight depression, and the spot will feel a bit tender. Press here firmly for 20 seconds, release, and repeat several times.

AROMATHERAPY FOR BETTER SLEEP

4 drops of neroli oil
3 drops of Roman chamomile oil
3 drops lavender oil
2 ounces unscented natural oil

Before doing the above touch remedies, rub a few drops of this aromatherapy blend

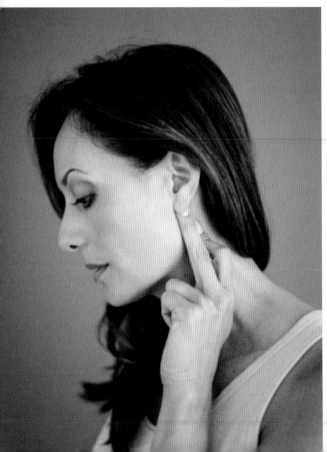

between your fingertips. Take a few deep inhalations of the scent on your fingertips, and then proceed with the remedies.

Aging Beautifully

Touch has a memory.
—JOHN KEATS

I know that every woman would love to age gracefully, without wrinkles, discoloration, or sagginess to mar a glowing complexion and without cellulite or extra weight that requires jeans in the next size up. Heck, there's an entire industry built around injectable fillers, laser treatments, and fad diets that will supposedly turn back the clock. However, if the idea of a needle injecting god-knows-what into your face or a tube sucking fat out of your butt does not appeal to you, I have several *natural* remedies that will soften the signs of aging and help you look and feel younger (and less stressed!). I've been using these techniques since I was in my twenties, and I swear *they work*!

For your face, there's the Facial Rejuvenation Acupressure Remedy based on an acupuncture facelift that's been used by the Chinese since the Sung Dynasty (960–1279 CE). Back then, acupuncture was used for cosmetic purposes on the empress (and the emperor's concubines) to improve circulation and stimulate the body's natural anti-aging powers. Today, it's an effective nonsurgical and painless way to lessen the appearance of fine lines as well as deeper wrinkles. In a study reported in the *International Journal of Clinical Acupuncture,* out of 300 participants, 270 perceived a marked decrease of facial wrinkles after just one treatment, and their skin felt firmer to the touch, with improved elasticity.[13]

And don't worry—you're not going to be sticking needles into your face! The Facial Rejuvenation Remedy uses acupressure (fingers, not needles) to stimulate specific points on the face to encourage the movement of blood and the production of collagen. This, in turn, nourishes, rehydrates, and tones the skin and reduces the appearance of facial wrinkles. You can do this technique anywhere, even in your car at a stoplight, so try it! I think you'll like it.

For the body, there's the Cellulite-Blaster Lymphatic Massage Remedy, which uses lymphatic massage to lessen that darn cottage-cheese look, and the Leg Lifter Swedish Massage Remedy, which uses Swedish massage to firm up your thighs. Every woman deserves to look and feel beautiful, and these touch remedies are a natural way to help you get there. Give yourself a few minutes of touch therapy every day, and you'll find yourself glowing inside and out!

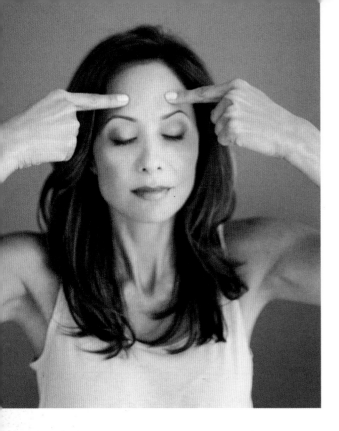

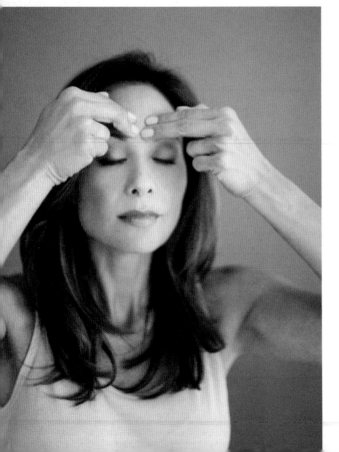

FACIAL REJUVENATION ACUPRESSURE REMEDY

....

Every woman deserves a natural way to look refreshed and youthful! This remedy is based on a traditional Chinese acupuncture facial that involves sticking many needles into your face. Now, I've actually had this lovely treatment, needles and all, and despite the panic attack I had when I looked into the mirror and saw Pinhead from the *Hellraiser* series, I admit the results were pretty remarkable. But it's definitely not for everyone! Instead, this Facial Rejuvenation Acupressure Remedy is a less invasive but very effective technique that anyone can do at home to help reduce wrinkles and puffiness. It'll increase circulation to your face for a healthy glow and can help you look five to ten years younger when done regularly. I recommend doing it at least once a week. Add this remedy to your beauty routine and you'll have gorgeous glowing skin in just a few weeks!

1. *"Yang White" (GB14) point:* Place the tips of your index fingers ½ inch above the center of each eyebrow. With medium pressure massage 10 circles to your right (clockwise). Hold for 5 seconds, and then repeat 10 more circles. Repeat a total of three times.

2. *"Third Eye" point:* Place both index fingers right between your eyebrows in the place where the bridge of the nose meets the center of the forehead. Press firmly for 60 seconds, then release. Repeat two times. This stimulates the pituitary gland, the main endocrine gland that helps to enhance the condition of the skin all over the body.

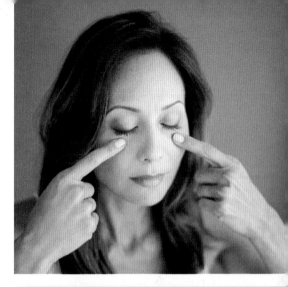

3. *"Four Whites" (ST2) point:* Place your index fingers 1 finger-width below the lower ridge of the eye socket, right below the iris and near the cheekbone, on both sides of your face. Press this point firmly for 60 seconds, release, and repeat two times. This can help reduce blemishes and acne.

4. *"Facial Beauty" (ST3) point:* Move your index fingers down about 1 inch to the bottom of the cheekbone, directly below the pupil. Press for 60 seconds, release, and repeat two times. Stimulating this area improves circulation and relieves acne, blemishes, and saggy cheeks.

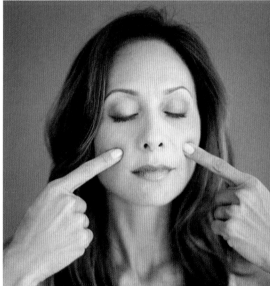

5. *"Heavenly Pillar" (B10) points:* Finally, bring your index and middle fingers to the back of your neck and press about ½ inch below the base of your skull on the muscles ½ inch outward on either side of the spine. These points help to balance the thyroid gland. Stimulating them improves your complexion and relieves stress, eye-strain, stiff necks, and sore throats.

CELLULITE-BLASTER LYMPHATIC MASSAGE REMEDY

"Cell-u-leet," as the French, who coined the term, say (also known as orange-peel or cottage-cheese skin), is a *bummer* for 80 to 90 percent of all women. No matter how much expensive cream or self-tanner you apply, those darn dimples won't go away! To set the record straight, cellulite is not a type of fat; it's a description of that dimpled look caused by fat deposits just below the surface of the skin. Although the exact causes are not known,

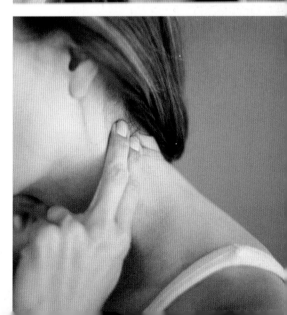

medical theories say that it's related to genetics, hormones, poor diet, lifestyle factors (smoking, no exercise, sitting or standing a lot), and, believe it or not, tight clothing that limits blood flow.

Sadly, there's no real cure for cellulite, but there are ways to make it less noticeable. This anti-cellulite remedy is a very effective lymphatic "skin-rolling" massage technique that will increase the blood circulation to the affected areas and activate the lymphatic system. It'll help you fight the good fight against cellulite and make you feel good enough to get into your skimpiest dress or even your bikini! For visible results, I recommend doing this remedy for at least 5 minutes every day for each problem area.

This massage technique is not relaxing in the slightest. In fact, it feels kind of strange and make take a few minutes to get used to. However, it's completely safe, not at all painful, and it beats liposuction by a long shot!

1. Warm some oil in your hands. Choose the area you'd like to work on (thighs, tummy, hips, etc.) and warm up the skin by kneading. Pick up as much of the skin as you can with the palms of your hands, and massage as if you were kneading bread. This increases circulation. Do this for 60 seconds.

2. Pinch an area of skin between your thumbs and forefingers and slowly pull your hands away from the body, rubbing deep into the tissue to help break up and smooth cellulite. You'll feel the skin separate from the fascia underneath. Hold the skin between your fingers and make a slight pinching motion as you gently roll the skin in one direction. Try to maintain the same amount of skin between your fingers as you move your fingers ½ inch down and repeat the pinch and skin rolling. Do this until you've covered the entire body part.

3. Place one hand on the skin to hold the area taut and then use the heel of your other hand to rub in circular motions, 10 seconds in each direction. Begin at the bottom of the affected area and slowly work up toward the heart. Try to cover the entire area.

4. Finish by applying long, smooth strokes with the palms of both hands moving toward the heart. It's extremely important to drink lots of water after this kind of lymphatic massage, as it releases various toxins trapped in the tissue into the bloodstream.

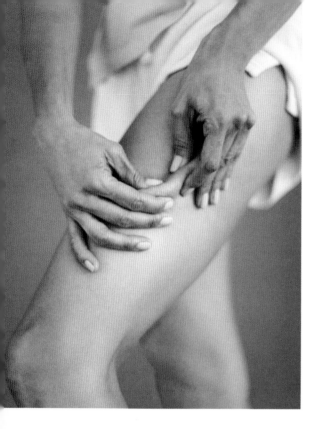

AROMATHERAPY FOR CELLULITE

....

20 drops juniper oil
10 drops rosemary oil
10 drops geranium oil
10 drops grapefruit oil
4 ounces unscented natural oil

Blend the oils together and inhale the scent. Place a small amount on the palm of one hand, then rub your hands together. Spread the oil onto the body part you're focusing on and firmly massage it into your skin. These powerful detoxifying oils will stimulate your skin and you will feel some cool, tingling sensations.

LEG FIRMER SWEDISH MASSAGE REMEDY

....

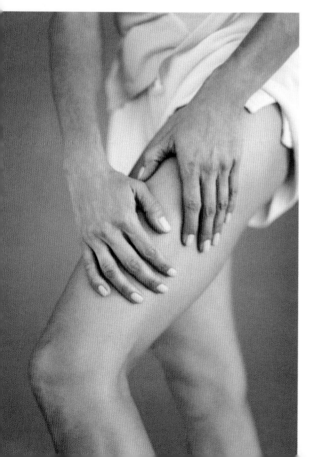

Everyone wants firm, flab-free legs, right? Not only can lean legs help you lead an active lifestyle; they can help you look healthy and sexy! Although exercise and diet are essential to firming up your legs, Swedish massage, which consists of long gliding strokes in the direction of the heart, can help boost the circulation in your legs, flush out toxins (lactic acid) in the legs that cause swelling and muscle soreness, and improve muscle tone. On top of all that, Swedish massage is extremely relaxing. Whether you prefer massage that is slow and gentle or vigorous and invigorating, this remedy will relieve stress and shape up those lower limbs!

I. Sit comfortably so you can reach your entire leg. I prefer to sit on a bed with my leg outstretched in front of me. Don't forget the towel underneath! Warm some oil in your hands. Beginning at your ankle, apply firm pressure and stroke both hands around the leg and all the way up to the top of the thigh. Do this several times to cover the entire leg.

2. Focus on your thigh by using the palms of both hands to stroke upward from the knee to the thigh, one hand at a time. Continue to apply firm pressure, alternating hand over hand. Do this for 15 seconds on the front of the thigh, and 15 seconds on the back of the thigh.

3. Place your palms on each side of your leg and stroke both hands up to the top of the thigh several times. This encourages the blood flow toward the heart.

4. Finish with three or four long strokes with both hands beginning at the ankle and stroking up the entire leg to the top of the thigh.

5. Repeat on the other leg.

Menopause and PMS Management

When I turned forty-five, a lovely friend with good intentions enthusiastically explained to me what I could expect in the upcoming decade. "Honey," she said, "menopause is puberty's evil older sister, and she's on her way to visit!" I'll never forget it. By the year 2020, the number of women older than age fifty-one (the average age of menopause) is expected to be more than fifty million in the United States.[14] So if you're in that group, you've got some company!

With this many women entering "the change," as it's commonly called, it's time for everyone to realize that suffering in silence is *out* and taking care of yourself is *in*. Whether you suffer from headaches, hot flashes, night sweats, bloating, exhaustion, insomnia, weight gain, mood swings, memory problems, breast tenderness, lack of libido, or all of the above, there's help for you in the form of new treatment options and natural therapies. Touch therapy can help you help yourself at a time when your body often calls for instant relief.

Menopause is a natural event that normally occurs to *all* women ages forty-five to fifty-five, and there are many ways to make this phase of life, and the years leading up to it, more pleasant. Menopause is defined as the absence of menstrual periods for one year or more, but the decreasing levels of estrogen produced by the ovaries can cause unpleasant symptoms that may begin earlier than you'd expect. The good news is that there are several touch-therapy techniques you can use to ease the symptoms of menopause and give yourself some relief.

If you're in or anywhere near "the change," I suggest trying these easy, natural techniques, treating mood swings, hot flashes and night sweats, and memory and concentration issues, that have been used by women around the world for centuries to help relieve the symptoms of menopause. And keep in mind this mantra from one of my dear menopausal friends: "I'm still hot. It just comes in flashes now!"

MOOD SWINGS REFLEXOLOGY REMEDY

During menopause, mood swings can be a daily, if not hourly, occurrence! In addition to anxiety, anger, and depression, if you feel as though you want to tear someone's head off one minute and then find yourself dissolving in a puddle of tears the next, you know what I'm talking about. Similar to PMS, hormonal changes can wreak havoc on your emotional state and negatively affect your body's endorphin levels. Furthermore, insomnia and night sweats—two other common problems during menopause—can lead to moodiness and irritability. Studies show massage can help reduce PMS-like symptoms such as pain, water retention, and mood swings.[15]

A British study found that foot reflexology reduced menopausal symptoms of anxiety, depression, hot flushes, and night sweats by approximately 30 to 50 percent. And in a study from China, daily reflexology sessions of 30 minutes for sixty days helped 40 percent of the menopausal women in the study fully recover (symptoms disappeared, no relapse at two months), and 48 percent of the women significantly recover (symptoms disappeared, relapsed at two months but disappeared with more treatment).[16]

As for PMS, a study published in *Obstetrics and Gynecology* showed that women who received reflexology had a 46 percent reduction of premenstrual symptoms, including headaches, backaches, insomnia, menstrual cramps, anxiety, and mood swings.[17] Now that's encouraging!

To get your moods under control, try this simple reflexology remedy that can easily be done several times a day. I recommend doing it once in the morning and once in the evening for maximum effectiveness.

I. *Reproductive organs reflex area:* Sit comfortably so that you can reach your ankles. Place your index finger on the back of your ankle and your fourth finger on your anklebone. Your middle finger will fall in the hollow just below the anklebone on the inside of the ankle. Once you've found that spot, locate the same spot on the outside of the ankle. These two areas are the reflex areas to the reproductive organs. Place your thumb on one of

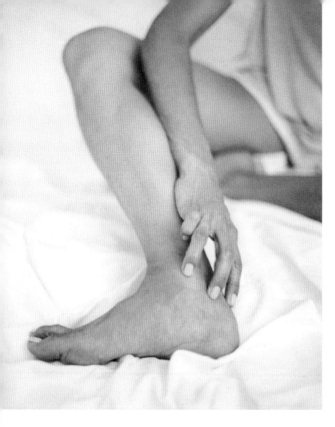

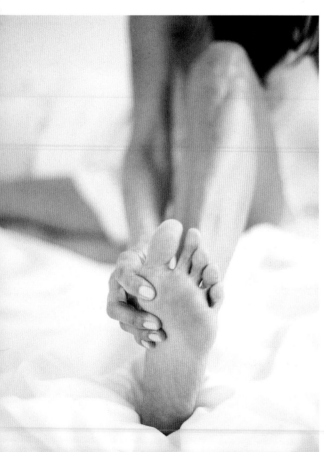

the hollow spots and your middle finger on the other hollow spot. With firm but gentle pressure, make small circles in one direction for 10 seconds and then hold for 5 seconds. Release and repeat several times. This is a direct energy channel to the reproductive organs, and pressing this area can relieve congestion and make you feel better.

2. *Brain reflex area:* On both feet, pinch the fleshy part of the big toe behind the nail to stimulate the reflex area to the brain. Make small circles in one direction for 10 seconds, and then reverse directions for 10 seconds. This can calm an overactive mind and help you to think more clearly. Pressing here stimulates the pituitary hypothalamus and pineal areas and helps to control hot flashes and circulation.

3. *Thyroid and neck reflex area:* Press your thumb into and make small circles along the crease at the base of the big toe and in the pad below the big toe on the ball of the foot. This stimulates the reflex areas to the thyroid, which regulates the body's hormone levels, and the neck. This can help balance your emotions and ease anxiety.

AROMATHERAPY FOR MENOPAUSE

....

6 drops lemon oil
5 drops geranium oil
1 drop jasmine oil
2 ounces unscented natural oil

These essential oils can calm and relax you and help you sleep better; all are safe to use during pregnancy.

HOT-FLASH AND NIGHT-SWEAT
ACUPRESSURE REMEDY
....

Hot flashes can leave you looking and feeling like a red, hot, sweaty mess in less than a minute. They're the most frequent symptom of menopause, and they happen in more than two-thirds of women during perimenopause and almost all women with induced menopause or premature menopause. (I actually have a friend who carries a battery-operated fan with her at all times!) Night sweats, which are severe hot flashes that occur while you're sleeping, can wake you up in the middle of the night, drench your clothes and sheets, and leave you cold and clammy with a pounding heart.

Although the exact cause of hot flashes is not known, it's believed to be a complex interaction that involves decreasing estrogen and progesterone levels, the hypothalamus (a region of the brain that regulates body temperature), norepinephrine (a key brain chemical), and the body's blood vessels and sweat glands. The sudden feeling of heat can lead to a rapid heart rate and cause red blotches to appear on the chest, back, and arms followed by heavy sweating and cold shivers to cool the body back down. Awesome. The takeaway is this: hot flashes and night sweats are simply annoying and must be stopped. Try this acupressure technique two to three times every day to help keep those pesky hot flashes and night sweats away!

Researchers from the North American Menopause Society (NAMS) analyzed twelve studies and found that acupuncture has the power to reduce hot-flash frequency and severity and other menopausal symptoms. They found menopausal women between the ages of forty and sixty had lessened the frequency and severity of their hot flashes for as long as three months after an acupuncture treatment.[18] Now, I know you can't stick needles into yourself, but you can apply pressure to the exact same areas for effective results.

1. *"Yin Cleft" (H6) point:* With your thumb, apply firm and steady pressure to the point on the topside of the wrist, about ½ inch above the wrist crease and ½ inch from the outer edge of the pinkie-finger side of the wrist. Press and hold for 10 seconds. Make small circles in one direction and then the other for another 10 seconds. Release and repeat on the other hand. Stimulating this point can help with hot flashes accompanied by sweating, and night sweats. You can do this several times throughout the day.

2. *"Three Yin Crossing" (SP6) point:* To find the acupressure point, place your pinkie finger at the top of the ankle bone on the inside of your ankle

(your pinkie should be just touching the ankle bone). Where your index finger lands along the side of the shinbone, feel for a soft depression just off the bone on the side closer to the back of your leg. Once you've found this point, use your index finger or thumb to apply pressure. Press and hold firmly for 10 seconds to relieve and prevent hot flashes. Make small circles in one direction and then the other for another 10 seconds. Repeat on the other leg. This is one of the most potent points for women's health, as it strengthens the spleen and kidneys, nourishes the blood, regulates the uterus, relieves pain, calms the mind, and promotes the smooth flow of energy, or *chi*.

3. *"Great Stream" (K3) point:* Place your fourth finger on the inside of your anklebone and your index finger on your Achilles tendon. The area where your middle finger lands should be the depression near the anklebone, at the same level with the tip of the anklebone. Press your middle finger firmly on this area for 20 seconds, and then make small circles in one direction, then the other. This invigorates and strengthens the kidneys and regulates the uterus.

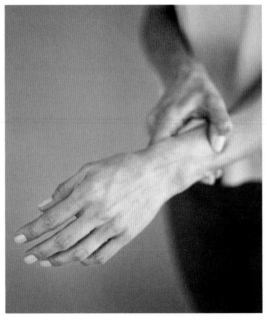

Yin Cleft (H6) Point

4. *"Bubbling Spring" (K1) point:* Press your thumb on the sole of the foot, between the second and third toes, at the point that's approximately one-third of the distance between the bottom of the toes and the heel. Again, press and hold firmly for 10 seconds, and then make small circles in one direction and then the other for another 10 seconds. Repeat on the other foot. This point helps hot flashes and night sweats. It also helps to strengthen the kidneys, which, according to Chinese medical theory, are associated with water and counteract fire and heat from the heart or liver. The kidneys are also associated with reproduction and growth. During menopause, your kidney energy can be weak, as your reproductive ability ends.

MEMORY AND CONCENTRATION
ACUPRESSURE REMEDY

In a disordered mind, as in a disordered body, soundness of health is impossible.
—CICERO

Brain fog and short-term memory loss are extremely common and frustrating during menopause, as clarity of mind is something no one wants to lose. If you can't remember where you put your keys or what you're supposed to get at the grocery store when you get there, you're not alone! For many years health-care professionals didn't take these problems seriously, and many women felt as if they were going crazy when they were told to accept forgetfulness and the lack of focus as part of growing older. But new research proves that it's not all in your head! In a study published in the journal *Menopause,* researchers concluded: "The memory problems experienced by women in their 40s and 50s as they approach and go through menopause are undeniable, and they appear to be the most acute during the early period of post-menopause."[19]

Now that the health-care industry is paying attention, women can rest assured that these problems don't have to be permanent and can be helped by lifestyle changes (i.e., addressing stress and sleep issues) and beneficial therapies. This acupressure remedy can help jump-start your recovery to clear thinking and better memory and put an end to menopause's absent-minded haze!

1. *"Heavenly Pillar" (B10) point:* Place your middle and index fingers on the back of your neck, about 1½ inches below the base of the skull and

1½ inches away from the spine, on both sides. Press and massage circles in one direction and then the other for 2 minutes. This can help relieve stress, burnout, and unclear thinking. Repeat three times every day to relax your neck and encourage better circulation to your brain.

2. *"Three Mile" (ST36) point:* On both legs, press the middle and index fingers of each hand into the area about 2 inches below your kneecap and ½ inch away from the shinbone. You can do both legs at once or one leg at a time. To check whether you're on the right spot, move your foot up and down and a muscle will move under your finger. Apply firm pressure here for 2 minutes three times a day. Stimulating this point on both legs will strengthen your mind and help you gain mental clarity.

3. *"Bigger Rushing" (LV3) point:* Press your thumb or index finger on the top of each foot, about 2 inches from the bottom of the big toe, on the point where the big toe and the second toe bones meet. Apply firm pressure for 2 minutes. Do this three times each day on each foot to improve poor concentration and encourage clear thinking and focus. This helps clear congestion in the liver meridian.

touch remedies soften the signs of aging and help you look and feel younger.

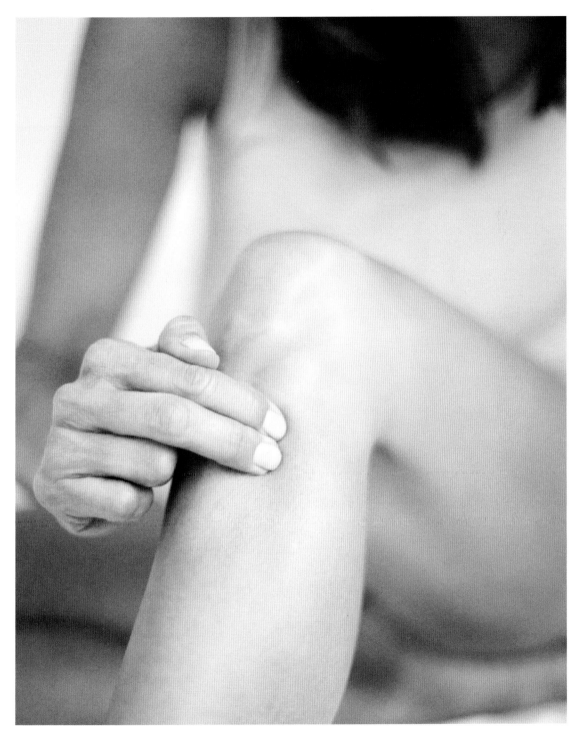

Three Mile Point

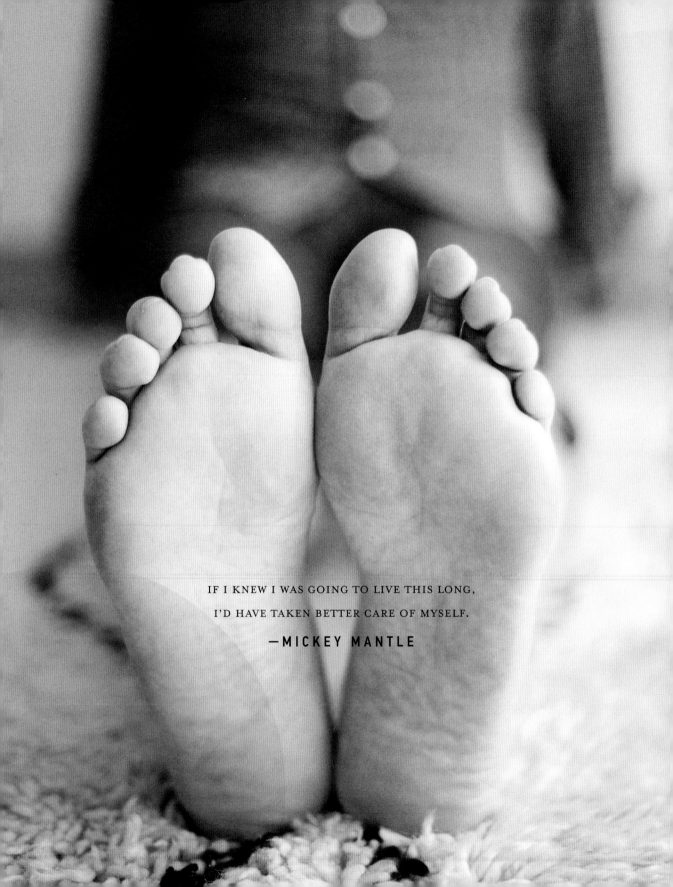

IF I KNEW I WAS GOING TO LIVE THIS LONG,
I'D HAVE TAKEN BETTER CARE OF MYSELF.
—MICKEY MANTLE

CHAPTER FIVE

Men's Remedies

Massage Away Your Problems

Men today are in need of some help when it comes to their health. Although most men will passionately debate this fact, ask doctors and they'll tell you: men, in general, are less healthy than women by practically any measure. It's true! Life expectancy for men is currently about seventy-five years, versus eighty years for women, and men are one and a half times more likely than women to die from heart disease, cancer, and respiratory diseases. Additionally, in our culture many men suffer from physical and emotional *touch isolation,* meaning they're cut off from platonic human physical contact that's proven to reduce stress, encourage self-esteem, enhance personal connections, and build a sense of community.[1] As a mom to three boys, I know this needs to *change*. Men, it's time to start treating yourselves with more kindness! And women, we need to encourage the men in our lives to start now!

First off, men need to learn to take better care of themselves. Many conditions that plague men are preventable, and men have the power to improve their health if they embrace a more mindful and proactive attitude. What's been holding them back? Their attitude toward health care. Unlike women, who learn to practice preventative health care at an early age (e.g., annual ob/gyn visits beginning at age thirteen), most men have a pattern of reactive care. They seek medical attention only when something is serious rather than investing in preventative measures earlier on. In fact, men are 40 percent more likely to skip recommended health screenings and make half as many visits to their doctors as women. Men are also plagued by character traits—including emotional suppression, aggression, and risk taking—that are associated with fewer visits to health-care providers and higher rates of injury and disease.[2]

For instance, my own lovely husband fell off a balcony during a raucous high-school spring break and completely tore off his pinkie finger. Yes, he fell to the ground two floors below, but his pinkie stayed on the balcony, which wasn't good news for a football tight end and aspiring professional musician! Luckily, a quick-thinking friend put the pinkie on ice, and doctors were able to reattach it, but the damage was done!

As for stress, although men and women may be equally stressed, men deal with it differently. Women are inclined to talk about how they're feeling physically and emotionally, but men notoriously have trouble putting their feelings into words, so they keep things bottled up inside. As a result, they're more subject to the damages of stress. Additionally, some men respond to illness and stress with denial, because to them those things represent weakness or vulnerability, and they're not motivated to seek help. So by the time a man finally seeks help, the problem is more difficult to treat. According to Rick Kellerman, president of the American Academy of Family Physicians (AAFP), "One of the biggest obstacles to improving the health of men is *men* themselves. They don't make their health a priority."[3] Perhaps for real change to occur in the way men approach their own health care, they may just have to get sick and tired of being sick and tired!

The second obstacle men must overcome in order to live a healthier lifestyle is lack of touch—something that adds more stress to an already stressful life. Although most of us are unaware of it, most men in American culture suffer from platonic (nonsexual) touch deprivation, which damages them physically and emotionally. This means that men are missing gentle, loving, compassionate touch (and, of course, the physical and emotional benefits that come with it) from friends, family, and even strangers that is not sexual in nature in any way. And, yes, that kind of touch does exist!

In reality, one of the reasons for this "touch isolation" is that most men in our culture are uncomfortable with physical contact with anyone other than their significant other (whether female or male) for fear that it will be misinterpreted as sexual in nature. Although it's common etiquette for men in other cultures to kiss and hug when greeting both men and women, it's rare for men in our culture to have close physical contact with anyone without assuming a sexual intention. In Asia and India, for example, it's normal for heterosexual men to walk down the street holding hands in friendship. In America, though, hand holding between male friends is a rare thing, as homophobia has driven it out of typical acceptable social mores.

So how did this come about? In our culture, an inappropriate, oversexualized view of human touch, combined with generations of puritanical sexual shaming, has taught boys to keep their hands to themselves, as all touch may be seen as sexual. Boys, whose parents typically put an end to physical affection when puberty approaches, often grow up with limited physical contact and end up channeling their need for touch into the occasional roughhousing with friends or aggression on the basketball court. Not surprisingly, boys who are raised with minimal touch grow up to be men who refrain from touching, holding hands, and hugging because they're just not accustomed to it. Yet they still crave touch and must channel that need somewhere.

According to Myles D. Spar, Director of Integrative Medicine at Venice Family Clinic and author of *Integrative Men's Health,* "Men have to develop safe, contained, and culturally appropriate outlets for their need to be physically bonded to each other." Dr. Spar described a cartoon to me that illustrates men's need for platonic contact with other men as a way to cement a bond and receive support. In the cartoon, two men are playing football and celebrating a good play by high-fiving and then half embracing and patting each other on the back; the caption reads: "Straight men develop elaborate rituals as excuses for touching one another."[4] As psychologist Dacher Keltner notes, "Touch is the original contact high."[5]

Unfortunately, the vast world of platonic human touch for men in our culture has been reduced to the exclusive domain of one person (the spouse or significant other) and is generally sexually connected.[6] Dr. Spar states, "American cultural mores have loaded touch from either gender with men as potentially sexual, overshadowing the power of touch to help form bonds, provide comfort, and reinforce emotional connection with guilt and self-consciousness. Men in the United States feel constrained in their ability to engage in any physical contact."[7]

Men are uncomfortable with platonic touch on so many fronts: with women because it may be sexually construed, with men because of our homophobic culture, and with children because they don't want to risk being seen as a sexual predator. In addition, men are less likely to reach out and touch someone else because, in our touch-averse culture, they fear rejection as well as appearing "soft" rather than tough or manly. Sadly, this leaves most men, especially those without a significant other, truly touch deprived.

Yet there is hope! According to Dr. Spar, "The more American men can learn to touch and feel touched, the healthier they will be."[8] In other words, by overcoming their fear of touch and learning how to express emotions and affection through touch as well as accepting touch, men can live healthier lives and potentially transform our culture's view of touch for our children. And I can tell you, as a mom who smothers her boys with love and physical affection on a daily basis, this is a particularly inspiring goal.

The good news is that if men can learn to be in tune with their body, take care of it proactively, *and* integrate more healthy touch into their day-to-day routine, the quality of their life can dramatically improve. If men can recognize a problem (instead of ignoring the signs), seek support, and find ways to treat it early on, through self-care techniques as well as medical intervention, they'll feel better and live longer.

Gentlemen, by learning how to use these touch-therapy techniques on yourselves, I promise you will become more in tune with your own bodies and see how comforting as well as therapeutic touch can be. And hopefully, this will encourage you to be more receptive to touch from others. Ladies, as partners, mothers, friends, or family members, you can help by using touch-therapy remedies not only to heal, but also to introduce touch in a nonthreatening way to the men in your life who may otherwise be averse to touch.

In this chapter, I've put together my most effective touch-therapy techniques specifically for common male issues, which all men can do to help themselves before the problems become chronic and damaging. There are DIY solutions for back and muscle aches, prostate and urinary problems, and erectile dysfunction. These remedies can help men be proactive, enhance their sense of touch, and improve their own health!

So women, if you're reading this and I've struck a chord, bookmark this chapter and pass it on to the man or men in your life who could use some help. And for all you men out there, I encourage you to take a good look at your health, schedule your preventive doctor appointments regularly, and try these touch-therapy remedies today!

We have to frame health-care seeking as an act of self-reliance. The message should be that taking charge of your health is what it means to be a real man.

—Dr. W. Hammond[9]

WEEKEND WARRIOR DEEP-TISSUE REMEDY

You can't be sedentary from Monday to Friday, then play football or run a marathon on the weekend, and expect to be okay! People who try to make up for inactivity during the week with long bouts of strenuous activity on the weekends are bound to get injured. Most commonly, weekend warriors are formerly active people over age thirty whose work and family obligations prevent weekday exercise, so they cram it into the weekend. Weekend warriors are not only sports enthusiasts, but also home-improvement enthusiasts who overuse their muscles for extended periods of time and aren't prepared for that increased level of activity. The most common injury is muscle strain.

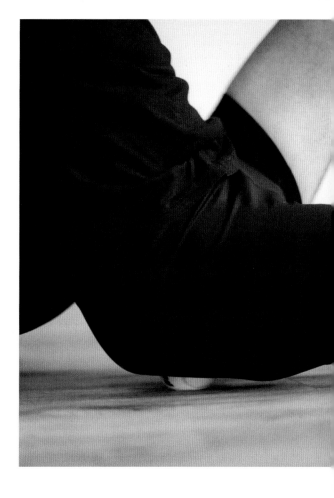

But relief is here! A recent NIH study found that kneading sore muscles after exercise actually turns off genes associated with inflammation and turns on genes that help muscles heal. Another study found that using SMR (self-myofascial release techniques) on people with short hamstrings resulted in immediate increases in flexibility of the hamstring.[10]

Here's a great remedy you can do yourself to help release tension, ease pain, speed recovery, and make yourself feel so much better. This deep-tissue rolling technique uses a foam roller, PVC pipe, or tennis ball, placed underneath your muscles to give you a much deeper massage than you can get from simply rubbing them. This is also a form of self-myofascial release, in which you can help break down adhesions or "knots" in your muscles, so they can heal properly. I love it (and I'm no weekend warrior)!

1. *Sore butt:* Sit on the floor with one leg bent and the other leg extended in front of you. Place the tennis ball under your butt on the side with the straight leg. Keeping both hands on the floor to help your body move on the ball, allow your body weight to relax onto the ball. Use your bent leg to slowly move your body back and forth, and side to side, over the ball. Roll slowly and gently, and pause on any tender areas until you can feel them release. Repeat on the other side.

2. *Sore calf muscles:* Sit on the floor with one leg bent and the other extended in front of you. Place the foam roller or PVC pipe under your calf (perpendicular to the leg) and let the weight of your leg relax over it. Keep your hands on the floor, slightly behind your back, and slowly inch your body backward, so that the roller glides all the way down your calf to your ankle. Then slowly inch your body forward so that the roller glides up the leg to your knee. Repeat several times in each direction to relax the calf muscles, and then switch legs. (You could also do this with a tennis ball, but it's harder to control a ball than a longer roller or pipe.)

3. *Sore hamstrings:* Sit in the same position on the floor with one leg bent and the other extended in front of you. Place the roller or pipe under your leg (perpendicular to the leg), just above the knee, and let your body weight relax over it. With hands on the floor to support you, slowly inch yourself forward, so the roller glides all the way up the hamstring, and then slowly inch in the other direction. Repeat several times, and then switch legs. You can also try this with both legs on the roller, but this requires you to hold up more of your weight on your hands. I like massaging one leg at a time, because you can better control the pressure on your leg by leaning from side to side.

4. *Sore shoulders and back:* Lie on the floor (knees bent, feet on the floor) and place a tennis ball under the area that is tense. Allow your body weight to relax over the ball for a few seconds, and then move your body so that the ball massages that area. You can also use the roller by placing it under your back, near your lower back, and slowly inch your body, so that the roller rolls all the way up your spine to your neck, and back down. Repeat several times. To relieve shoulder tension, turn the roller so that it is parallel to the spine and place it between shoulder blade and spine. (You can also do this with a tennis ball.) Slowly move your body, so the roller rolls over the shoulder area (*not* over the spine). Try opening your arm out on the floor and then folding it over your chest as you roll back and forth slowly. This is my favorite stress reliever!

PROSTATE OR URINARY PROBLEM
REFLEXOLOGY REMEDY

....

Unfortunately, an enlarged prostate, as well as the annoying and sometimes painful urinary problems that accompany it, is a problem most men will confront in their lifetime. More than 50 percent of men in their sixties have symptoms of an enlarged prostate (a condition known as benign prostatic hyperplasia, or BPH) and that number rises to as much as 90 percent when men reach their seventies and eighties. Prostate infections are relatively common, usually occurring in men after age thirty, and the prostate is the number-one cancer spot in a man's body.[11]

The good news is there are many things you can do to keep the prostate healthy, and it's important to discuss the options with your physician. Reflexology has been shown to be effective in improving the symptoms of prostate disease. A study on reflexology from Denmark found that out of 46 participants, 65 percent experienced a reduction in their need to urinate, 67 percent experienced better bladder pressure, 60 percent experienced overall improvement in their general condition, and 80 percent experienced reduced sexual problems. Researchers concluded that reflexology can help prostate problems, as improvements were noted in all categories.[12]

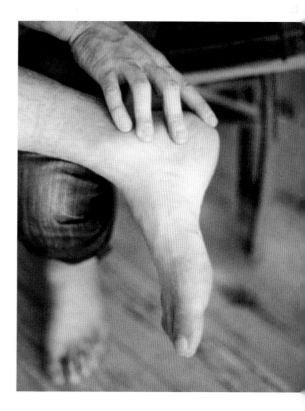

At home, try this self-reflexology technique that improves circulation and energy flow to the prostate and kidneys to keep them as strong and healthy as they can be.

1. *Prostate reflex area:* Sit in a chair and cross your right foot over your knee, so you can reach your ankle. With your right hand, place your fourth finger on your ankle bone and your index finger on your Achilles tendon. Your middle finger should fall into the indentation just below the anklebone. This is the reflex area to the prostate gland. Apply firm pressure for a few seconds, then make small circles in one direction for 1 minute and then in the other direction for 1 minute. Stimulating this area can open the energy pathways to the prostate and relieve any

congestion that could cause problems. Repeat on the other ankle.

2. *Kidney reflex area:* Place your thumbs just below the center of the sole of your foot. Press firmly for 10 seconds; then make small circles in one direction for 1 minute and then the other for 1 minute. Stimulating the reflex area to the kidneys improves the energy in the nerve pathway and strengthens the urinary system. Repeat on the other foot.

3. Do twice every day for maximum effectiveness.

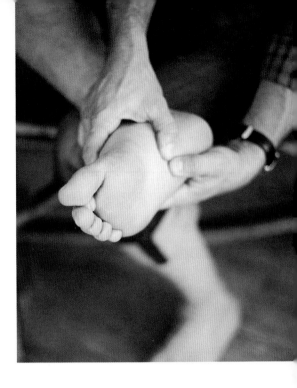

ERECTILE DYSFUNCTION ACUPRESSURE REMEDY

Erectile dysfunction (ED) is one of the most common male sexual problems, affecting an estimated 30 million men in the United States and approximately 140 million men worldwide. This number could be even higher since many men with erectile dysfunction are often embarrassed to come forward and seek help for their condition. At least 50 percent of men in the United States experience some form of sexual dysfunction at some point in their lives.[13] According to the NIH, approximately 5 percent of forty-year-old men and between 15 to 25 percent of sixty-five-year-old men experience ED on a long-term basis.[14] Occasionally, younger men may experience ED, which can occur for a variety of reasons, such as exhaustion or too much alcohol. As men get older, impotence becomes more common.

Fortunately, today there are many different ways ED can be treated, managed, and even reversed. In a study from China, reflexology was found to be as effective as traditional Chinese medicine for treatment of male sex-related problems. In the study, 37 men with sexual dysfunction were randomly assigned to two groups: one group was treated with daily 30-minute foot reflexology sessions, and the other group was treated with traditional Chinese medicine. Treatments lasted at least one month. Both groups experienced almost the same results. The men in the reflexology treatment group experienced improvements of 87.5 percent for impotence and 100 percent for the other types of dysfunction, and the men in the traditional Chinese medicine group experienced improvements of 85.7 percent for impotence and 100 percent for the other types of dysfunction. The important difference between the groups that the researchers note is that reflexology had the advantages of being easy, inexpensive, and drug-free.[15]

If you experience erectile dysfunction, talk to your physician—and try this drug-free remedy at home to boost your energy and help resolve ED.

1. *"Sea of Vitality" (B23 and B47) points:* Sit in a chair and reach your hands behind your back. Place your thumbs on your lower back, on either side of the spine, about 2 finger-widths away from the spine. Bring your thumbs to waist level, which is in line with the belly button, and between the second and third lumbar vertebrae. Press firmly (B23) for 30 seconds, release, and then move your thumbs another 2 finger-widths away from the spine and ½ inch down. Press firmly (B47) for 30 seconds and release. Repeat both points. Do this twice each day to relieve sexual-reproductive problems, impotency, and premature ejaculation. *Caution:* If you have any back problems, use lighter pressure and do not press on damaged or painful discs or bones.

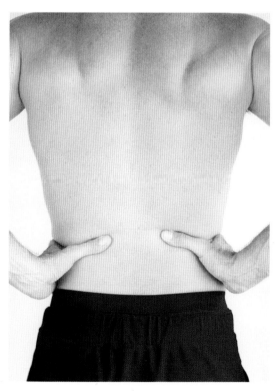

Sea of Vitality (B23)

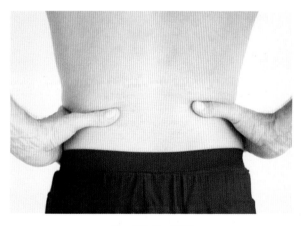

Sea of Vitality (B47)

2. *"Sea of Energy" (CV6) point:* Lie on the floor and place the index and middle fingers of either one hand or both hands (whichever you prefer) 3 finger-widths directly below the belly button. Press firmly for 20 seconds; then make small circles in one direction and then the other for 20 seconds. Stimulating this powerful acupressure point can help impotency.

3. *"Mansion Cottage" (SP13):* Lie on the floor and place your middle and index fingers on either side of your pelvis, on the area in the middle of the crease where the leg joins the upper body. Press firmly for 20 seconds; then make small circles in one direction and then the other for 20 seconds. Stimulating these powerful acupressure points can help impotency and abdominal discomforts.

4. *"Great Stream" (K3) point:* Sitting with one foot crossed over your other knee, place your middle and index fingers in the hollows on the inside of the foot, just below the anklebone. With firm but gentle pressure, make small circles here for 10 seconds, and then just hold for 5 seconds. Release, and repeat several times. Bingo! This is a direct energy channel to the testicles, prostate, and penis. You can't go wrong rubbing these two spots several times each day. Repeat on the other ankle.

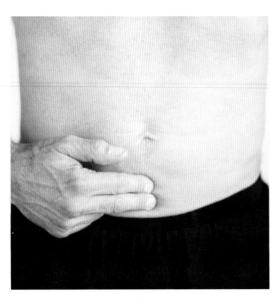

Sea of Energy

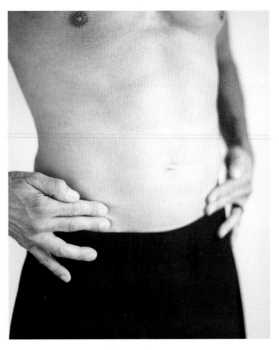

Mansion Cottage

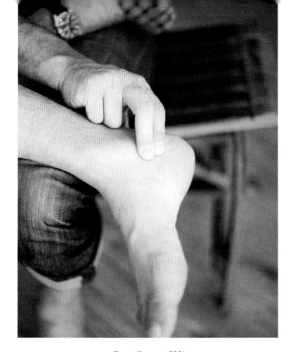

Great Stream (K3)

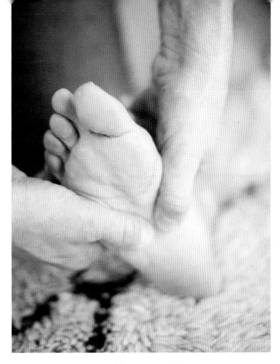

Bubbling Spring (K1)

5. *"Bubbling Spring" (K1) point:* Sit with one foot crossed over your knee and place your thumbs on the very center of your foot. Press firmly for 10 seconds; then make small circles in each direction for 20 seconds. Repeat on the other foot. According to traditional Chinese medicine, erectile dysfunction indicates that your kidney energy (or *chi*) is depleted, so stimulating this acupressure point to the kidneys can help ED.

AROMATHERAPY FOR MEN

> 4 drops peppermint oil
> 2 drops ginger oil
> 5 drops eucalyptus oil
> 2 ounces unscented natural oil

Most men like this aromatherapy blend because it's subtle and soothing for sore, tight muscles. Combine these oils and rub a few drops between your hands. Do the remedies as directed and the essential oils will enhance the results.

The way you think, the way you behave, the way you eat can influence your life by 30 to 50 years.

—DEEPAK CHOPRA

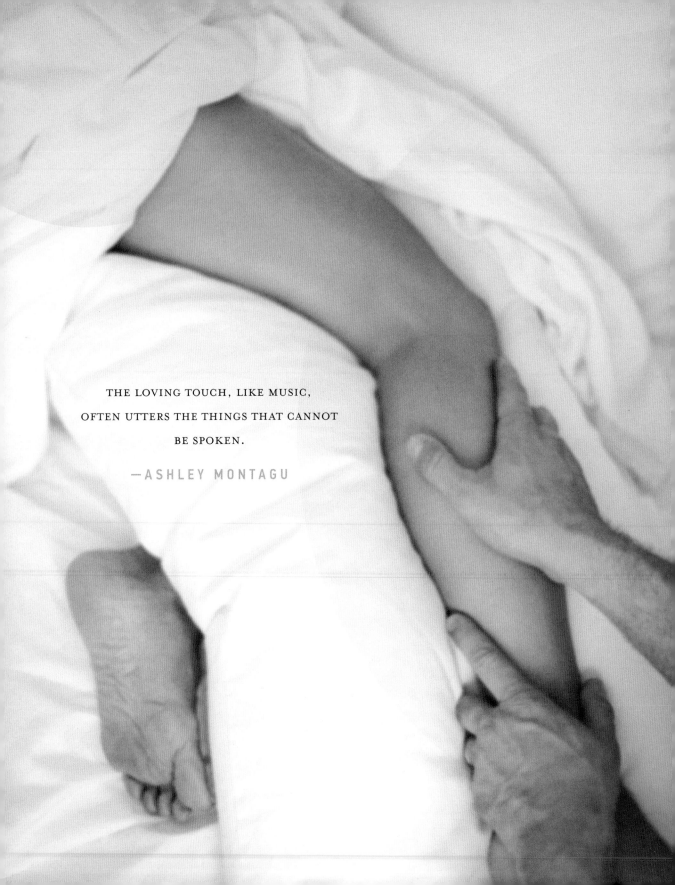

THE LOVING TOUCH, LIKE MUSIC,
OFTEN UTTERS THE THINGS THAT CANNOT
BE SPOKEN.

—ASHLEY MONTAGU

CHAPTER SIX

Hands on Your Partner

Enhance Intimacy with Touch

In my research for this book, when I interviewed friends (both straight and gay) about the importance of touch in relationships, every single person, male and female, quickly brought up *sex*. Well, this certainly opened up a can of worms:

"He wants to have sex all the time."

"How many times a week is normal?"

"Forget sex. I'm so tired I just want to be left alone."

"She never wants to have sex!"

Remarkably, not one person mentioned nonsexual touch until I brought it up. Certainly, touch is crucial in creating and strengthening romantic relationships, and it's no surprise that in our oversexualized culture most people automatically connect touch with sex. But studies now show that nonsexual touch is as important, if not more important, than sex to a healthy relationship. According to marriage experts, great sex isn't the key to a successful marriage;

rather, it's frequent caring touch that keeps couples happy![1] There's no better way to encourage more touch in your relationship than my touch-therapy remedies for partners, which are therapeutic, nurturing, bond enhancing, and above all stress relieving.

In relationships, touch really is the communication of love. It's a powerful way to express things that you may not be able to put into words. Momentary touches between you and your partner can communicate an even wider range of emotion than gestures or expressions and sometimes do so more quickly and accurately than words. Today, research proves that physical affection, both sexual and nonsexual, is highly connected to overall relationship and partner satisfaction.[2] Unlike words, which go to the brain's thinking center, touch goes directly to the body's emotional center. This encourages your partner to open up, let down protective walls, and express vulnerability, which is often difficult to do in our stress-filled world.[3]

I think most couples will agree that conflict resolution is much easier with more physical affection—and studies show that conflicts are resolved more easily with increased amounts of hugging, cuddling, holding, and kissing.[4] This kind of informal touch can enhance your relationship when things are good and repair it when things aren't so good. I know that when my husband and I are at odds, we stay far away from each other, as if there's a negatively charged energy field between us. However, all it takes is for one of us to reach out—maybe my hand on his neck or his arm around my shoulder—and the tension subsides. The problem itself may not have gone away, but at least we've connected on a sensory level.

Whether we're aware of it or not, everyone needs more touch than we're getting. The question is, in a relationship how much touch is enough? There's no proven scientific answer for this, as everyone is different, and thresholds for the amount of touch you desire to give and receive change on a daily basis. Although you may think you touch your partner often, it's interesting to note that, compared to those in the rest of the world, American couples are far behind in the frequency with which they touch each other. As I mentioned in Chapter 1, in a well-known study on how many times couples from different countries touched each other while sitting at a café, researchers found that, in a one-hour period, in Puerto Rico couples touched each other 180 times, in Paris 110 times, and in Florida twice.[5] *Only twice!!* But really, who's to say how many times you should touch your partner, especially sitting at a café? The point is that compared to people in other cultures, American couples are indeed touch deprived. Just the fact that we have a cuddling convention ("Cuddle Con"), companies that throw "cuddling parties" (Cuddleparty.com), and "cuddling spas," such as Cuddle Up to Me in Portland, Oregon, where people actually pay to get professionally cuddled, is proof that many Americans are craving touch.[6]

There are so many rewards to increasing the amount of comforting, nonsexual touch in your relationship. First and foremost, not only does it feel good; it's physically beneficial. Hugging, hand-holding, cuddling, and, yes, touch therapy all promote the release of the feel-good hormone oxytocin into the bloodstream and lower the stress hormone cortisol. This creates a feeling of calm that's been linked to increased trust, empathy, and bonding, which are all necessary things for a relationship. Studies show that oxytocin, also known as "nature's love glue," makes us more sympathetic, supportive, and open with our feelings. It's also linked to the longevity of a relationship, as couples with higher levels of oxytocin remained together longer and were more attuned to each other than those with lower levels.[7]

In a study at Brigham Young University, researchers found that couples may be able to enhance one another's health by being more physically affectionate with one another. They compared couples who underwent training in neck and shoulder massage as well as "listening touch" (which involves increasing awareness of the partner's mood by touching his or her neck, shoulders, and hands) with couples who did not learn these techniques and did not change their normal behavior. After four weeks, during which half of the couples practiced the touch techniques at home for 30 minutes three times a week, they found that couples who practiced the touch techniques had higher oxytocin levels, while their levels of alpha amylase, a stress indicator, were reduced.

In addition, they found that among men in the touched group, blood pressure was reduced after the four weeks. The researchers stated, "Our data suggest that warm partner contact may be particularly cardio-protective for men. . . . These findings may help us better understand the protective mechanisms of positive marital interactions in the prevention of stress-related diseases."[8] In other words, this may be one of the reasons that people with permanent partners or spouses live longer than those who live alone![9] Another study showed that touch between partners is related to lower blood pressure for women, for those who received more hugs from their partner had significantly lower blood pressure levels than those women who were not hugged by their partner.[10]

Truth be told, women aren't the only ones who crave nonsexual touch from their partner. According to a British survey of two thousand men, 67 percent of the men questioned said they wanted more cuddling in bed.[11] Other studies indicate that men who did not receive "affective affirmation"

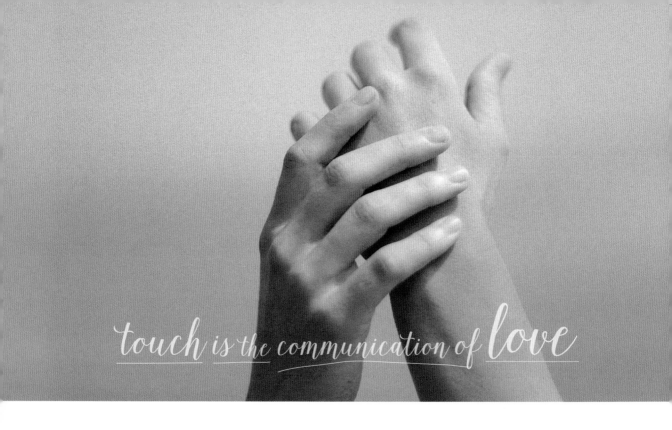

touch is the communication of love

in the form of physical (nonsexual) touch from their wives were two times more likely to divorce over time.[12] Partners who touch each other frequently are more satisfied with their relationship[13] and reported better psychological well-being six months later than partners who did not.[14] Perhaps most important, touch can help partners de-stress and get into a better mood, which everyone needs after a long, hard day.

In our touch-deprived culture, so many women complain that their relationship lacks intimacy. I promise that if you can find ways to bring more touch into your lives on a daily basis, intimacy will grow. Sex may get all the attention in the media, but it's really *touch* that will nurture and strengthen a healthy connection between you and your partner. It can make your partner feel valued, cared for, and above all loved. And you too will reap the reciprocal benefits of touch.

In this chapter you'll find valuable touch remedies that everyone can do to connect, communicate, and de-stress. I've used these remedies on my husband for years, and although he uses the excuse that, since I'm the expert, I should be the one doing the massaging, he's actually become pretty skilled in the techniques too. I guarantee that doing just one of these remedies will bring you closer and make you feel more connected in less time (and for less money!) than it would take to see a therapist. And don't wait until your partner is aching, in pain, or overly stressed-out to use these remedies. I recommend using them as often as you can, every day if possible. Your partner will thank you, and together you'll reap the benefits of soothing, stress-relieving, healing touch.

The remedies include:

- Intimacy Acupressure Remedy, to stimulate the body's erogenous zones, boost libido, and improve intimacy in relationships
- Back and Shoulder Deep-Tissue Remedy, deep pressure for maximum relief
- 5-Minute Reflexology Remedy, a reflexology routine to relax and connect
- Swedish Massage Remedy, a full-body massage for partners
- Thai Massage Remedy, partner massage techniques to de-stress

PARTNERS INTIMACY ACUPRESSURE REMEDY

Let's face it. No two people have the same level of libido at the same time. *Ever.* In relationships, one of the most common struggles is a difference in sexual desire and how to manage this energetic disparity, so that both partners are happy and satisfied. Although many women think that a man's libido is purely physical while a woman's is more emotional, that's not true. There are physical and emotional components to libido in both sexes. Although sexual appetite is directly related to diet, sleep patterns, hormonal deficiencies, and stress levels, it's also very much psychological. Unfortunately, sexual dysfunction is very common for both men and women. So if your urge to "get it on" has gotten up and gone, it may be comforting to know that you're not alone! The reality is that approximately 43 percent of American women and 31 percent of American men report having sexual issues.[15]

Results from a preliminary study suggest that acupressure can help reduce sexual dysfunction in women.[16] Another study suggests that acupuncture can help treat psychologically induced erectile dysfunction in men (relax—the prick points are all in the back!).[17] Whether you have a sexual issue or you just want to spice things up, this simple acupressure remedy is something that partners can do together to get in the mood, strengthen your sex drives, and bring passion back into your lives. Go ahead; try this remedy today. It's great foreplay as well as a soothing way to connect with your partner every day!

1. Press each of these points firmly for 10 seconds; then make small circles in one direction for 10 seconds and then in the other for another 10 seconds. Do this on both hands.

> *"Spirit Gate" (H7) point:* Located on the inside of the wrist, near the pinkie side, about 2 inches below the crease where the hand meets the wrist, this point can relieve anxiety, insomnia, and depression. It's believed that when this gate is open, you will have love, joy, and fun in your life.

> *"Rushing Door" (SP12) points:* Located in the pelvic area, in the middle of the crease where the leg joins the trunk of the body, on the left and the right, these two points are particularly good for relieving impotency, menstrual cramps, and abdominal discomfort.

> *"Mansion Cottage" (SP13) points:* Located in the pelvic area, about 3 finger-widths above the "Rushing Door" points, these points can increase a woman's sexual response and enhance sensations in the genitals.

> *"Bubbling Spring" (K1) point:* Located on the center of the sole of the foot, at the base of the ball of the foot, between the pads, this point can stimulate sexual energy.

2. *Bonus reflexology points:* Although this is an acupressure remedy, you can take advantage of some reflexology points here too. Place your thumb and middle fingers on the "hot spots" on the inside and outside of the ankle, in the hollow just below the anklebone, on both feet. These are powerful reflexology points that are direct energy channels to the uterus and vagina for women and the testicles and penis for men. Stimulating these points can boost your libido, ignite passion, and help your partner get in a sexy mood.

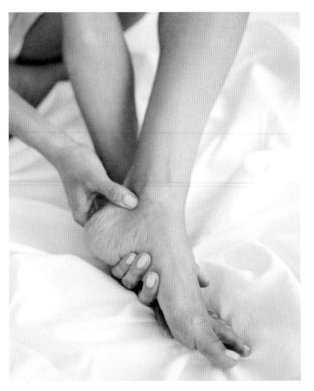

Hot Spots

PARTNERS BACK AND SHOULDER
DEEP-TISSUE REMEDY

If your partner works out a lot or just happens to carry a lot of stress in the back and shoulders, these deep-tissue techniques will work wonders to dissolve tension and relieve pain. Many people think that you have to be super-strong or physically large to give a good deep massage, but I can tell you that there are techniques that can help anyone, even very petite women, get deep into muscles without having to strain or use muscle strength. It's really all about manipulating your own body weight, no matter what size you are, and using gravity to your advantage. I'm 5 foot 5 and 110 pounds, and my husband is 6 foot 4 and 225 pounds, yet I can easily give him a very deep massage with hardly any effort at all. Conversely, my husband can give me a great massage without hurting me by simply backing off and not putting his full weight on me. With a little practice, you'll see that deep-tissue massage does not depend on your size, but rather how you shift your body weight around. If you or your partner suffers from knotted-up shoulders or a tight back, try this deep-tissue neck and shoulder remedy. I guarantee you will not be disappointed.

TOUCH IS A POWERFUL WAY TO EXPRESS WHAT YOU MAY NOT BE ABLE TO PUT INTO WORDS.

1. Always remember to communicate with your partner and ask if the pressure is okay. It's better to start with medium pressure and slowly adjust for deeper pressure by leaning your body weight toward your partner rather than leaning in too deeply in the beginning.

2. *Tight shoulders and upper back:* Have your partner sit in a chair with a low back. Stand behind the chair, lean forward, and place your elbows on what I call the "sweet spots," which are located on both sides of the spine at the top of the trapezius. The spots are at the base of the neck, a few inches away from the spine on each side. They're often very tight and painful, because that's where the upper trapezius, rhomboids, and levator scapula come together. Keeping your arm bent, slowly

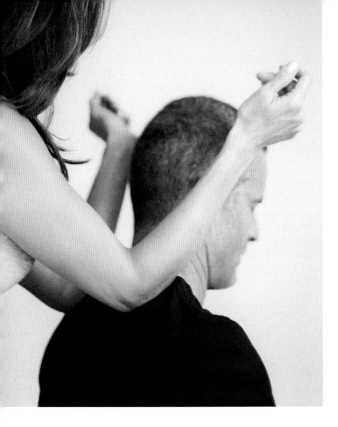

lean your body weight toward your partner, allowing your elbow to sink deeper in the muscle without using any force. You don't have to strain or use muscle strength to go deeper; just lean your body into it. Once the correct pressure is established, experiment with making small circles with your elbow and shifting your body weight so that your elbow position changes angles. This is an amazing stress reliever that everyone loves.

3. *Tight shoulders:* Sit in bed with your back against the bed frame and have your partner lie facedown on the bed in front of you (vertically), about 2 feet away from you. With shoes off (very important!), place your heels on your partner's shoulders, close to the neck, on either side of the head. There should be enough space between you, so your legs are comfortably bent. Slowly press one heel into the shoulder, then the other. If you want to get deeper into the shoulders simply push a little harder (sometimes it helps to hang on to the bed frame for leverage). Continue to alternate heels as you inch your heels out toward the edges of the shoulders, and then back in. Continually check in with your partner to make sure the pressure is okay.

4. *Tight back:* Have your partner lie facedown on the floor (on a carpet or yoga mat). Slowly and gently place your knees on your partner's buttocks and lower your weight so that you're kneeling on the gluteal muscles. Don't worry! The buttocks are well padded, with both fat and muscle, and they're one of the least

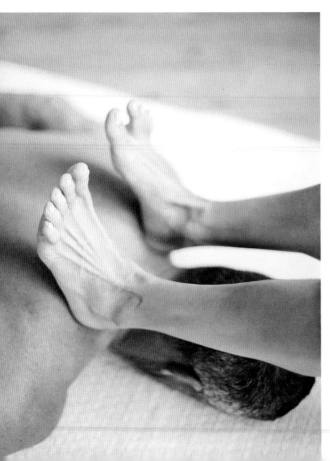

vulnerable places in the body, so you're not going to hurt anything. Shift your body left and right to stimulate circulation and apply deeper pressure. This not only releases the gluteal muscles; it also releases tightness in the lower back.

Next, lean forward and place your forearms on the muscles on either side of the spine. Shift your body weight forward as you alternate massaging each forearm up and down. Try to keep your arms on the muscles (called erector spinae) on either side of the spine. If the back is tight, it's easy for your arms to slide off. Do this for several minutes, experimenting with leaning your body weight forward and shifting from side to side.

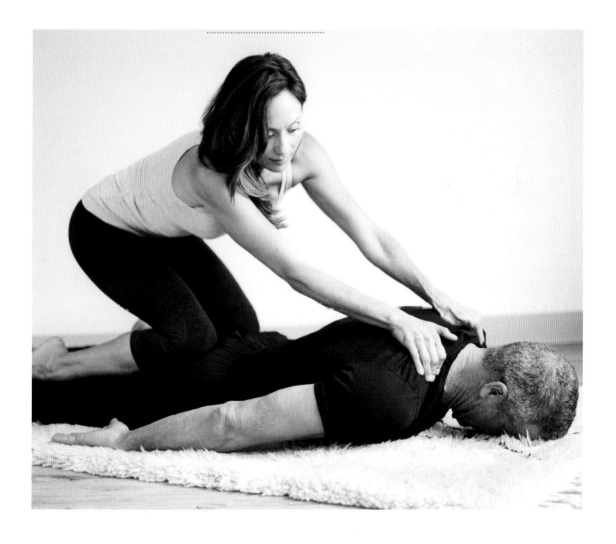

AROMATHERAPY FOR ROMANCE

SWEET AND SEXY

>   4 drops sandalwood oil
>   4 drops clary sage oil
>   2 drops orange oil
>   10 drops vanilla oil
>   2 ounces unscented natural oil

SULTRY AND SEXY

>   4 drops rose oil
>   6 drops sandalwood oil
>   2 ounces unscented natural oil

Blend the oils in either of the above recipes and rub a few drops between the palms of your hands. As your hands warm the oils, inhale the seductive aroma and then do the remedies on your partner.

PARTNERS 5-MINUTE REFLEXOLOGY REMEDY

The next time you're sitting on the couch with your partner, take 5 minutes and give each other a foot rub at the same time! I call it a "foot date," and you can actually relax your partner's entire body by simply massaging specific points on the soles of the feet. It's cheaper than a massage, and you both get to relax. All you have to do is grab a foot and get to work. (Socks can be on or off, although out of consideration for your loving partner, I do recommend washing your feet if you plan on taking socks off!) You can use oil or lotion if you choose, but it's not required. I actually like to use nothing, so that my fingers don't slip all over the foot.

Stimulating all the reflex points on both feet can encourage the entire body to come back into balance and stress to melt away. Once you get in the habit of doing this, you'll never stop. TV time can be transformed into relaxation time!

Play around with each of the areas to get to know what, how, and where your partner likes to be touched. After a bit of practice and good communication, you'll be able to really tune in to what your partner likes and needs.

I. *Getting ready:* Wash your hands so that they are clean and clear of any negative energy. Sit comfortably (opposite ends of a couch is perfect for this) and relax. Take your partner's feet in your hands and hold them for 10 seconds. This helps direct your focus to the feet and allows your partner to get used to the feeling of your touch. Take a deep breath, count to three, and exhale. If you are using lotion or oil, warm it in your hands and gently spread it over the top and the sole of each foot.

2. *Back stretch:* Bring both hands under the heels and pull them toward yourself, giving a slight stretch to your partner's lower back.

3. *Side-to-side ankle loosening:* Move your hands to one foot and place the outer edges of your hands at the heel. Move your hands from side to side to loosen the entire foot. Repeat on the other foot.

4. *Ankle rotations:* Bring one hand underneath to support the heel of one foot and rotate the ankle in one direction a couple of times, and then in the other. Repeat on the other foot.

5. *Achilles tendon stretch:* Gently push the toes back to release the arch of one foot, and then bring the toes forward, stretching the top of the foot. Next, flex the foot backward and then pull the toes toward you. Repeat. Then do the stretch twice on the other foot.

6. *Solar plexus relaxer:* Hold both of your thumbs at the solar plexus point, which is in the middle of the sole of the foot. This reflex point can relax and calm the entire body. Press for 10 seconds, release, and repeat. Then do the other foot.

7. *Thumb-walking:* Holding the first foot in one hand, use your other hand to thumb-walk up the foot. Place the thumb of your other hand on the heel at the inner edge of the foot and apply pressure as you gently inch your thumb up the foot toward the toes. When you reach the toes, bring your thumb back to the heel, move over about ¼ inch, and again thumb-walk up to the top of the toes. Repeat until you reach the outer edge of the foot. This allows you to stimulate every part of the body. Repeat on the other foot.

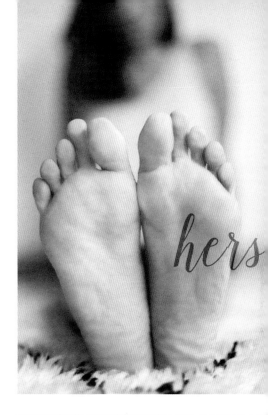

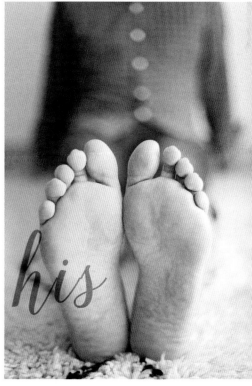

8. *Relaxing the back:* Use your thumb to make small circles on the inner edge of the first foot, starting at the heel and moving up to the bottom of the big toe. Repeat on the other foot. This relaxes the entire back.

9. *Calming the mind:* Pinch the fleshy part of the big toe between your thumb and index finger to stimulate the reflex area to the brain. Then do this on the other foot.

10. *Rolling the toes:* Many people find the toes very sensitive. Take each toe, one at a time, between your thumb and index finger, and slowly roll it back and forth. Try to move your fingers around the entire toe, so that you stimulate the whole toe. The area between the toes, close to the crease, is very sensitive in a lot of people. If your partner enjoys this, spend extra time applying light pressure there. Do the toes on the other foot.

11. *Stimulating the sexy areas:* Use your thumb and middle finger to make small circles on the inside and outside of the ankle, in the hollow just below the anklebone, on both feet.

12. *Feathering:* For a happy ending, finish by lightly brushing your fingertips from the tips of the toes to the heel, several times, on both feet.

NOTE: *As you work on each area, feel for "grainy" areas or places where the feet are tender. Grainy or tender areas are clues to energy blockages and potential "problem areas." Spend extra time on these areas, as they need it the most!*

PARTNERS FULL-BODY SWEDISH MASSAGE REMEDY

This is the ultimate partner remedy, a full-body massage in the privacy and comfort of your own home. Who doesn't want that? Swedish massage is a great way to build intimacy and closeness with your partner as well as relieve your partner's physical and mental stress. Unlike deep-tissue massage, which can be painful at times, Swedish massage is pure relaxation and soothing pleasure all the way. Studies suggest that a single session of Swedish massage therapy produces measurable biological effects, including decreases in cortisol and increases in lymphocytes, and these findings may have implications for managing inflammatory and autoimmune conditions.[18]

In another study, researchers measured immune function in healthy adults who got either a 45-minute Swedish massage or 45 minutes of lighter touch. The massaged group had substantially more white blood cells—including natural killer cells, which help the body fight viruses and other pathogens—and fewer types of inflammatory cytokines associated with autoimmune diseases.[19] In addition, research published in *Military Medicine* reports that military veterans indicated significant reductions in ratings of anxiety, worry, depression, and physical pain after massage from their partners. Analysis also suggests declining levels of tension and irritability following massage.[20]

Rather than go into too many technical details, I'm going to explain one basic stroke, the effleurage, which you can use on all parts of the body. *Effleurage* is a French word meaning "to skim" or "to touch lightly on," and that's exactly what you'll do. You'll use the palms of your hands and a little oil or lotion to lightly glide over your partner's entire body, stimulating nerve endings and relaxing muscles. Basically, an effleurage is a long, flowing motion using very slight pressure for upward strokes, then lighter pressure on the way back down. I like to think of the shape of the stroke as an elongated heart. You bring your hands straight up together then separate them as if you were drawing the top of a heart, and glide them back down to come together. That's all there is to it.

All you have to do is follow the steps below and let your hands guide you. Really, as long as you touch your partner gently and

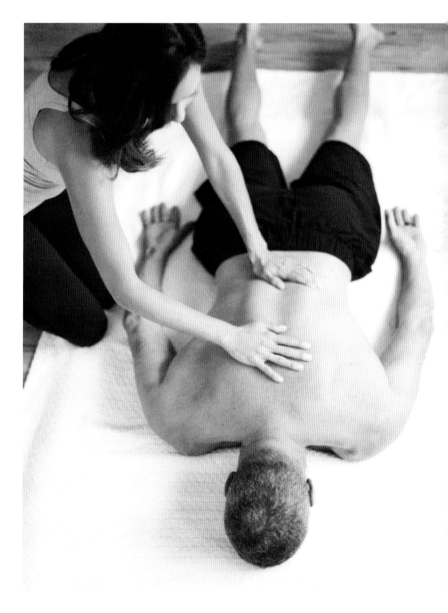

lovingly, you can't do anything wrong! Massage one part of the body or the entire body. Either way you're going to make your partner very, very happy!

1. *Back:* Place a towel on a bed (so you don't stain the sheets with oil) and have your partner lie facedown with the head turned to one side. Cover the legs with another towel or sheet to keep them warm. Warm some oil or lotion in your hands and begin with the back. Place your hands on the lower back and effleurage from the lower back to the upper back. Repeat as many times as you want, trying to touch the entire back.

2. *Legs and feet:* Cover your partner's back and legs with a towel or sheet to stay warm and move down to the feet. Uncover one leg (keeping the other leg warm under the towel or sheet). Use the same effleurage stroke beginning at the foot, moving all the way up the back of the leg to the top of the thigh, and then back down. Repeat several times. Then cover that leg, and repeat on the other leg.

3. *Top of legs:* Have your partner turn over and cover the torso, keeping one leg uncovered. Effleurage several times from the foot to the top of the thigh and back down. Cover that leg, uncover the other leg, and repeat.

4. *Arms:* Cover up the legs and uncover one arm. Effleurage from the hand to the top of the shoulder and back down. Do this several times, and then do the same for the other arm.

5. *Neck:* Make sure your partner is covered and warm. Reposition yourself so you're at your partner's head facing toward the feet. Reach your hands under the neck and place your fingertips on either side of the spine. Gently pull upward, starting from the base of the neck and moving up to the ridge at the base of the skull. Do this several times. Then reach one hand under the neck, at a slight angle, and pull back, so the head turns to one side. Then reach the other hand under the neck and pull back, so that the head turns from side to side. Alternate hands slowly, so the head turns back and forth and the neck is relaxed.

6. *Head:* Finally, bring your fingertips to your partner's head and massage small circles all over the scalp. Try to cover the entire scalp.

7. Voilà! You're done. Your turn!

PARTNERS THAI MASSAGE REMEDY

Thai massage is my absolute favorite kind of massage to give because, selfishly, I know I'm going to get as much out of it as I give. Developed in Thailand (obviously), this technique uses passive stretching and gentle pressure along the body's energy lines to increase flexibility, relieve muscle tension, and balance the body's energy systems. It's relaxing and energizing for both receiver and giver.

Thai massage is often referred to as partner massage or yoga therapy, because there's active engagement and communication between the giver and the receiver, and the giver uses his or her whole body (hands, knees, legs, and feet) to move the partner into a series of yogalike stretches. It's sort of like doing yoga without having to do the work. Unlike other touch-therapy techniques in which there's more skin-to-skin contact and the receiver is encouraged to zone out and relax, this technique requires the receiver to keep clothes on (to ease moving the body into different positions) and to actively participate. Because of this interaction, even though both partners remain fully clothed, I feel that Thai massage is actually more intimate than a traditional Swedish massage.

So if you're looking for a technique that will encourage your partner to relax and zone out, this is not the remedy. Try the Swedish massage remedy instead. However, if you want to try something that will relax muscles and energize both of you, this is the ticket! Here are the Thai massage techniques (or poses) that women and men of all sizes and strengths can do at home with their partner, safely and easily, for maximum health benefits:

The *Back Press* opens the shoulder and chest areas.

The *Cobra* stretches the middle and upper back and opens the chest and shoulder areas.

The *Down Dog* relaxes tight hamstrings and relieves back tension.

The *Warrior* relaxes tight hamstrings and relieves back tension.

In a study on Thai massage and pain threshold and headache intensity, researchers found that Thai massage could increase "pressure pain threshold" and reduce headache intensity, suggesting that it's a possible alternative treatment for chronic headaches.[21] In another study on Thai massage and pain, muscle tension, and anxiety in patients with scapulocostal syndrome (which is pain in the back and shoulder that may involve other parts of the arms or chest), researchers found that Thai massage could be an effective alternative treatment.[22] In a study of Thai massage and osteoarthritis of the knee (a common form of arthritis), researchers found that Thai massage (in combination with a Thai herbal compress) was as effective as oral ibuprofen after three weeks of treatment.[23]

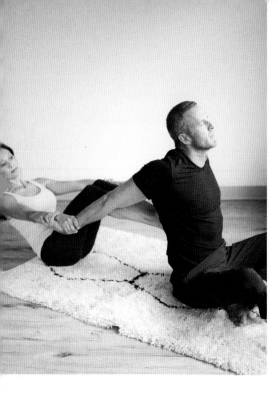

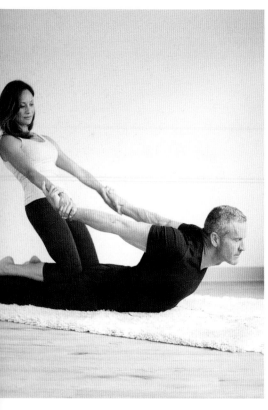

1. *Back Press:* Sit on the floor with your legs straight out in front of you, and have your partner sit in front of you but facing away from you, in the same position. (Alternatively, your partner can sit in a bent-knee, cross-legged position if it's more comfortable.) Position yourself so that you can comfortably place the soles of your feet (shoeless, of course) on your partner's lower back, on either side of the spine. Have your partner reach his or her arms back while you reach forward to take hold of each other's wrists. Next, apply pressure to the lower back with your feet and at the same time lean back slowly. Ask your partner how it feels and experiment moving your feet slightly up and down the back, keeping the pressure even on both feet. This gives a nice stretch to your partner's chest and upper back and your upper back. The more you lean back, the greater the stretch.

2. *Cobra:* Have your partner lie facedown on the floor. Slowly bring your knees down onto your partner's buttocks, so that the top of your knee is on the fleshy part of the buttocks and your shins are along the hamstrings (in effect, you are kneeling on your partner's buttocks and hamstrings). Reach down and take hold of your partner's forearms and tell your partner to grab your forearms. Very gently lean back. This gives a great stretch to your partner's chest, back, and shoulders as well as your upper back and your quads. The more you lean back, the greater the stretch. You can also lift your shins up and off the back of your partner's legs, which is a bit harder on your quadriceps, but it gives an extra stretch as you lean back. Don't let go of each other's forearms! Your knees give your partner's buttocks a gentle compression that feels so good. Ask your partner how the stretch feels and if you should go deeper. I like to do this a few times. In between cobras I let my partner relax on

the ground, while I lean forward and give a gentle squeeze to his shoulders.

3. *Down Dog:* Have your partner lie facedown on the floor. Begin by kneeling on your partner's buttocks. Slowly and gently place one foot and then the other onto his or her upper hamstrings and bring both of your hands onto the upper back on either side of the spine, so that you find yourself in a Down Dog position. Experiment with shifting your weight forward and back and moving your hands ups and down the back (always keeping your hands on the muscles on either side of the spine, *never* directly on the spine). This gives an amazing massage to your partner's back and hamstrings at the same time.

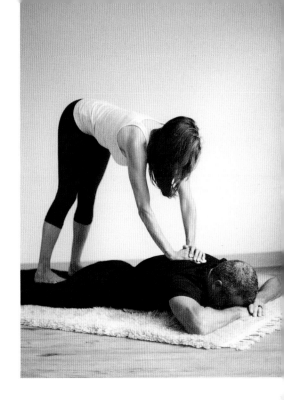

4. *Warrior:* If you and your partner are comfortable in the Down Dog position, this is the next step. Bring your right foot forward and place it to the right of the spine (again, *never* on the spine!). Keep your hands on your partner's back or, if you find it hard to balance, you can bring a chair close to you for stability. Gently ease your weight forward onto your right foot and back to your left foot, which should still be on your partner's left hamstring. You can experiment with moving your front right foot up and down the muscles on the side of the spine. This Warrior position is a great way to give a deep massage with hardly any effort on your part. Repeat on the other side. Most important, don't forget to communicate with your partner throughout this entire remedy and if your partner ever complains that it's uncomfortable, just get off his or her back (literally).

At the touch of love, everyone becomes a poet.

—PLATO

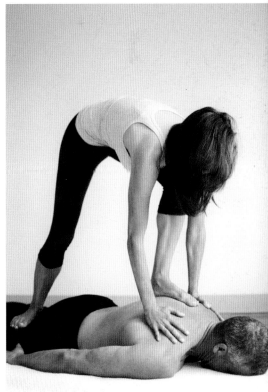

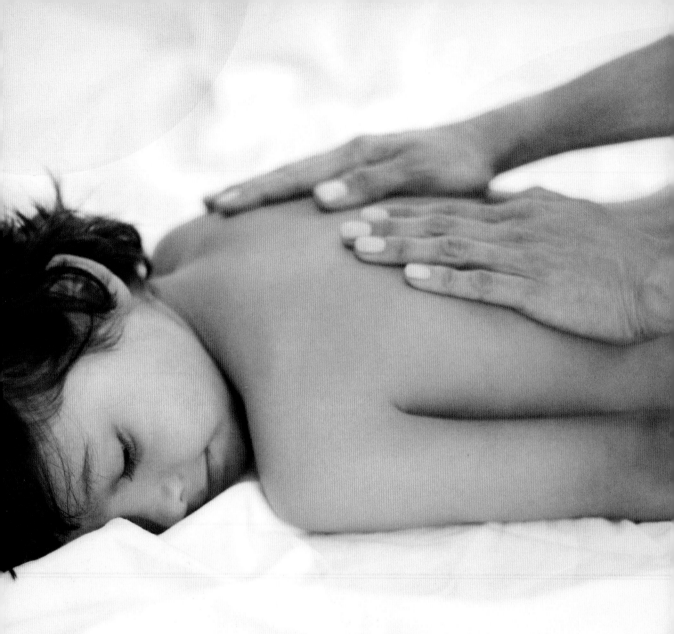

TO BE TENDER, LOVING, AND CARING, HUMAN BEINGS MUST BE TENDERLY LOVED

AND CARED FOR IN THE EARLIEST YEARS, FROM THE MOMENT THEY ARE BORN.

HELD IN THE ARMS OF THEIR MOTHERS, CARESSED, CUDDLED, AND COMFORTED.[1]

—ASHLEY MONTAGU

CHAPTER SEVEN

Calm Kids

Touch Remedies for Kids of All Ages

Have you ever seen a baby shift from fussy and restless to quiet and calm in seconds when her legs are massaged? Or a toddler in constant motion actually stop and lie still when you rub his back? Possibly even more powerful are the emotional turnarounds of moody, angst-ridden teenagers who finally begin to open up and communicate after a 5-minute foot massage, and the improvements in energy level of exhausted college students who learn to use self-massage as a tool for caring for themselves while away at school. Touch can truly have amazing effects on kids of all ages!

In both hospitals and homes, I've witnessed dramatic transformations in thousands of children using simple touch techniques that everyone can do. As a massage therapist, a certified infant massage instructor, and, most important, a mother, I know personally that touch is a powerful tool for parenting that has enormous benefits for both children and parents.

Research shows that touch is truly fundamental to human communication and bonding, and it's essential to a child's development, sense of well-being, and good health.[2] Touch therapy can help children who have difficulty sleeping, reduce anxiety, and improve a child's ability to focus and concentrate. It can also ease many physical and emotional symptoms associated with pediatric medical conditions. And yet studies show that American babies and children are among the least touched on earth.[3] I'm here to encourage all parents to start gentle touch therapy on their children from day one, or as close to day one as possible.

Babies need touch and attention in order to thrive. As they grow up, they continue to need regular touch and attention to become warm, caring, independent people. Researchers at Harvard University report that "physical contact and reassurance will make children more secure and better able to form adult relationships when they finally head out on their own."[4] American childrearing practices today are influenced by fears that children will grow up dependent, and some parents have a "let them cry" attitude toward their kids. There's a happy medium between the hands-off, "be independent" parenting style and the overprotective, helicopter parenting style, and daily touch is necessary and beneficial for both.

Most parents will do anything and everything to keep their children physically and emotionally healthy, and that includes keeping them as stress-free as possible. Touch can help reduce stress hormone levels, which in turn strengthens the immune system to help the body stay healthy and strong. What's more, children who learn to view touch in a positive way are more likely to grow up to be adults with healthy self-esteem, a sense of security, and proper boundaries for intimate relationships.[5]

I've watched many children who were massaged regularly throughout their childhood grow up to be the most balanced and confidant young adults I've ever met. While my three boys are still young, I try to massage them for at least a few minutes every day to relax their bodies and minds, release stress from the day, and nurture a close bond that I hope will continue as they grow up to be adults. Even though I can't control the stress that comes their way each day, as a parent I can help how they handle that stress, and that's something I wish I'd learned at an earlier age.

No matter how old your children are, they'll always be your babies, and touch can help you help them. In this chapter, I'll share my simple touch remedies for children of all ages, from newborns to young adults. The chapter is divided into 4 sections: "Babies," "Toddlers and Tikes," "Touchy Tweens and Teens," and "College Kids." In "Babies," you'll find simple, safe, and effective baby massage techniques to help soothe newborns to two-year-olds. In "Toddlers and Tikes," there are easy touch remedies to calm busy, nonstop toddlers and little kids. In "Touchy Tweens and Teens," you'll learn nonthreatening massage moves that will help you communicate and reconnect with hormone-fueled teenagers. Finally, in "College Kids," I'll share my favorite self-massage remedies to help college kids relax, focus, sleep, and manage their own stress levels.

Each touch-therapy remedy has helped me and my own family conquer stress, and I hope they'll do the same for you. I know how hard it is to raise kids, and my goal is to teach parents simple techniques to communicate peace and love—one child at a time. By focusing attention on your children and spending real quality time with them as you touch them, you'll be able to nurture their health and well-being at every different stage of life. To get started, all you need are your own two hands, and you're good to go!

Babies

The art of baby massage teaches parents how to give and receive nurturing.
—Dr. Tiffany Field

People often laugh with skepticism when I tell them that babies need massage. But when babies come out of a warm and very cozy womb, they are immediately bombarded with an overload of unfamiliar sensory stimulation, including the emotional energy of people around them, that they're unequipped to handle. So they react with tension and frustration by either crying or withdrawing, which is why many newborns fall asleep when they're in a noisy restaurant. White noise is actually a proven infant sleep aid. In an experimental study of newborns, 80 percent of infants assigned to hear playbacks of white noise fell asleep spontaneously within 5 minutes, while only 25 percent of control infants fell asleep spontaneously.[6]

Baby massage is a valuable tool for parents, because it helps your baby learn how to handle stimulation and stress and respond to it calmly. Since about 80 percent of a baby's communication is through body movement, touch is one of the most effective ways to communicate with your baby. I know that massaging my three babies from the day they were born helped me tune into their body language and interpret their moods and needs. When you get to know your baby's body, you'll have a good sense when something feels "off." For example, when you feel your baby's tummy and it's a bit harder than normal, you'll realize that gas bubbles may be causing irritability. You can then use specific massage techniques to help your baby release the gas.

touch is essential to a child's
development,
well-being, and health

Benefits

There's significant scientific evidence that regular massage gives your baby a physical, emotional, and intellectual advantage for a healthy childhood. Clinical studies led by Tiffany Field, at the University of Miami's Touch Research Institute, showed that:

> Babies who are massaged appear more active and alert and have faster neurological development than babies who are not massaged.

> Full-term babies who are massaged regularly cry less, experience less stress, enjoy better circulation and digestion, and develop stronger and healthier minds and bodies.

> Baby massage is especially helpful for premature babies! Twenty premature babies—massaged for 15 minutes, three times a day, for two weeks—gained 47 percent more weight than babies who were not massaged. They were also discharged six days earlier from the hospital, saving the hospital over $10,000 per infant.[7]

Once you understand the benefits of touch, I guarantee you'll want to massage your baby every single day. It's the greatest feeling in the world when a fussy baby calms down and stares into your eyes during a massage. You know that baby is tuning into the sensations from your hands and learning how to relax and "let go." There's really nothing more important than a healthy and happy baby. So enjoy this special time with your child, and touch your baby with your hands and your heart.

Babies benefit immensely from massage, which:

- Enhances communication and nurtures the parent–child bond
- Relaxes and soothes baby's nervous system
- Decreases the production of stress hormones
- Reduces fussiness and irritability
- Helps baby sleep longer and more soundly
- Strengthens and regulates baby's respiratory, circulatory, and gastro-intestinal functions
- Relieves gas and constipation
- Reduces colic
- Reduces pain associated with teething
- Improves baby's muscle tone and motor skills
- Promotes faster weight gain
- Enhances baby's sense of touch and provides a wealth of sensory experiences

- Promotes a healthy body image
- Helps separation anxiety for infants in day care
- Benefits premature babies who remain hospitalized
- Benefits special-needs infants whose mental, visual, hearing, or developmental impairments make bonding more difficult
- Stimulates the brain and contributes to mental growth and development[8]

Parents benefit from baby massage as well! For parents it:

- Promotes parent-child bonding
- Improves communication with baby
- Enhances intimacy, understanding, and parents' ability to nurture
- Increases parent confidence
- Decreases postpartum depression and nervousness (which can indirectly affect the baby's mood)
- Involves fathers in an intimate way
- Helps parents of premature and special-needs babies who remained in the hospital after birth reconnect
- Encourages a special, focused time for bonding and interaction
- Improves parental understanding of baby's nonverbal cues
- Increases the parent's ability to calm a stressful or sick child
- Helps parents with babies in day care
- Helps working moms reconnect with baby after a long day at work.[9]

FAQs

Why do babies need massage?

Because babies need touch! Massage provides the extra tactile stimulation babies need to release stress and relax their little bodies. Research shows that babies who are massaged have physical and emotional advantages over those who are not massaged.

When can I begin massaging my baby?

If your baby is healthy, you can begin gentle touch-therapy techniques (light touch with no pressure) on day one. At three weeks of age you can apply gentle pressure, which babies prefer over lighter touch.[10] Consult your physician if you have concerns.

How often should I massage and how long?

I recommend massaging every day, even if for just a few minutes. A 10- to 15-minute massage is the most beneficial, but go with the flow. If your baby's enjoying it, keep going. If not, then stop. When babies start moving around a lot, they may not lie still for more than a minute or two. But don't let that discourage you! Touching your baby with love for even 2 minutes can work wonders.

How much pressure should I use?

During the first few weeks of your baby's life, the massage you give should use very light pressure. At three weeks of age, you can apply more firm, yet gentle and soft pressure. If the pressure is too light, babies perceive it as tickling and are less receptive. According to Tiffany Field: "Although infants, particularly premature infants, for example, may seem to be fragile, some pressure is needed for the massage to be effective. In our review of the infant massage literature, we found that those who used light stroking did not report weight gain, for example, while those who used stroking with pressure reported weight gain."[11]

How can I tell if my baby likes it and if I should keep going or stop?

If your baby gets quiet, makes eye contact, or even smiles, the baby is probably enjoying your touch. If your baby pulls away, looks away, or starts to cry, that's a good indication that the baby doesn't want to be massaged. Sometimes babies get a little fussy when you begin, but will settle down once they get comfortable with your touch.

If you begin to massage and your baby resists or gets upset, continue momentarily to see if the baby is distracted or perhaps has gas. If the fussing continues, stop. You can try again later. Babies may cry at the start, and this is perfectly okay. Staying calm and relaxed yourself is important.

No matter what, do not force the massage. You want this experience to be positive for both you and your child, and your job is to help your baby feel safe and loved. If your baby is not into it, respect that and stop.

When's the best time of the day or night to massage my baby?

Anytime you want your baby to relax! I recommend doing it after a bath and before bedtime. But if your baby is learning to crawl or trying to stand, a leg massage or back massage during the day can relax the muscles that are working so hard to move the body weight around. Always wait at least 45 minutes after baby eats before massaging.

Is massage recommended for special-needs babies?

Absolutely. However, parents with special-needs babies should always consult a physician before massage. Your baby's response to massage may be different than what is outlined in this book because of special needs and challenges.

Where did baby massage come from?

Baby massage is one of the oldest healing arts and has been part of child-care traditions around the globe for centuries. Parents from countries with different cultural practices, such as India, Africa, Bali, and China, have passed their own baby-massage routines down through the generations. Here in the West, many hospitals are beginning to include massage in their neonatal programs.

The bond between a parent and child is one of the strongest and most important of all human attachments. All babies and mothers possess natural instincts that encourage the bonding process, and baby massage incorporates them all, including:

- *Touch:* Mothers instinctively stroke their babies after birth. Massage provides the tactile stimulation babies need to feel safe and secure.
- *Eye contact:* Newborns focus their eyes at about 7 to 12 inches, which is the ideal distance for face-to-face interaction during a massage.
- *Smell:* Newborns can detect the odor of their mother, which gives them a sense of security. When mothers are near their babies, they release the maternal hormones oxytocin, the "love hormone," and prolactin, which stimulates the production of milk. (This is why I suggest using unscented massage oil during the first two months, so as not to disturb baby's sense of smell.)
- *Sound of mother's voice:* Babies are attuned to the high-pitched tone that mothers often use, and they're capable of distinguishing the mother's voice from other voices beginning in the seventh month of pregnancy. Talking to baby during massage is extra comforting!

Daily Massage for All Babies from Day One

To prepare for baby massage, choose a *warm* and *quiet* room with dim lights (no harsh overhead lights shining into baby's eyes). Play only relaxing music, nothing loud or raucous, although silence is good too. Wash your hands, make sure your fingernails are not too long or sharp, and remove any jewelry with pointy or rough edges. Above all, relax—babies can sense if you're nervous or uncomfortable.

You'll need three to four towels, one or two for under baby, one for your hands, and another to quickly clean up the occasional "accident" (especially with boys!); a soft comforter or blanket; and unscented all-natural oil (I recommend sesame and almond oils). For the first two months, I recommend using only unscented oils so that the mother's own scent can reach the baby, which reinforces bonding. Later, you can enhance your massage with aromatherapy by adding 2 to 3 drops of a soothing essential oil to 2 ounces of an unscented natural oil base in a dark glass bottle (blue or amber) to maintain freshness. Aromatherapy can help calm babies who cry persistently or have difficulties with eating or sleeping.[12]

AROMATHERAPY FOR BABY MASSAGE

Lavender: a soothing, healing antiseptic oil

Roman chamomile: a calming, soothing oil, good for sensitive skin

Fir needle or cypress: a decongestant, great for when baby has a cold or cough

Sweet orange: a mood- and energy-lifting oil (promotes cheerfulness)

These are my top aromatherapy essential oils for massaging baby. Choose any one and add a few drops to 2 ounces of unscented natural oil. (Always add essential oils to a base, as essential oils are potent and can cause stinging and irritation if applied directly on the skin, especially for babies, who are supersensitive.) Apply a few drops of oil to the palm of one hand and rub your hands together to warm the oil. For baby massage, you want your hands to have enough oil on them to glide gently over baby's skin, but not so much that it's slippery and greasy. Less is better than more. Remember, you can always add a few more drops of oil to your hands but it's much harder to get rid of an oil slick!

RESEARCH SHOWS
REGULAR MASSAGE
GIVES YOUR BABY A
PHYSICAL, EMOTIONAL,
AND INTELLECTUAL
ADVANTAGE FOR A
HEALTHY CHILDHOOD.

Basic Positions for Baby Massage

Choose whichever position is most comfortable for you:

1. Sit cross-legged on the floor or bed. Place a towel (large enough to lay your baby on) in front of you. If you're on the floor, fold a comforter for extra padding and place the towel on it. Lay your baby on his or her back facing you, about an arm's length away.

2. If you prefer to stand, place your baby on a changing table or a table that's high enough so that you aren't slouching down too much and stand in front of him or her. Make sure you always have one hand on the baby for safety. *Never* leave baby unattended!

3. For newborns I recommend sitting on the floor with legs outstretched, knees slightly apart, heels together, and back against a wall or couch. Place a comforter and a towel on the floor between your legs, then place the baby on top facing you. This makes a kind of cradle between your legs that provides a sense of warmth and safety.

Tips to Keep in Mind

- Always warm oil in your own hands first. Never pour oil directly onto to the baby's skin.
- Do *not* give the baby a pacifier or bottle during massage.
- Only one person at a time should massage the baby.
- Try to maintain eye contact with the baby while you massage. Talking also helps the baby relax.
- There's no exact number of strokes that you should do for each part of the body. Trust your intuition and let your hands repeat the strokes as many times as your baby is comfortable with.
- If you massage one leg or foot, remember to do the other, so that baby doesn't feel out of balance; same with arms and hands.

Contraindications to Baby Massage

When *not* to massage a baby:

- *Illness:* Do not massage your baby if he or she is ill. Consult your physician before beginning massage.
- *Skin rashes and infections:* Do not massage over any areas that are irritated or infected.
- *Immunizations:* Wait at least one week after an immunization before massaging your baby. Avoid massaging directly on the injection area, which may still be sensitive.

- *Your mind-set:* Avoid massaging if you are ill, exhausted, or just not into it.

Massaging Preemies

Premature babies are very protective of their bodies and may be resistant to letting you massage them at first. Since preemies are too young for eye-to-eye contact, you have to rely on other cues. Oftentimes, hiccups may signal stress. If a baby begins to hiccup or withdraws from your touch, he or she may be overstimulated. To soothe the baby, try my calming techniques below. Always get your doctor's approval before massaging a preemie, as weight is a factor in safety.

How to Calm a Baby Before and During Massage

1. *The holding method:* If you sense that a baby is restless or not used to being touched, with baby lying in front of you, place your hands over baby's ears and head for 10 seconds. This gives baby time to feel the warmth of your hands and relax. You can also rest the palms of your hands on baby's legs, which seems to slow their movements. When you're both calm, you can start the massage.
2. *Arms and legs toward chest:* With baby lying front of you, gently cross baby's arms in front of the chest and, at the same time, bring baby's legs up to the chest. This is a more "organized state," one close to the fetal position, which babies find comforting. From here, let the baby open up when he or she is ready to relax.

The Sequence for a Full-Body Baby Massage

This is the sequence that I prefer to follow, but feel free to follow your intuition and let your baby's responses guide your routine. As you try the massage strokes on different parts of the body, you'll begin to develop your own intimate form of nonverbal communication with your child. Go with what your baby enjoys!

1. *Legs and feet:* These are the least vulnerable parts of the body and often the most receptive to massage early on.
2. *Arms and hands:* As your baby gets used to your touch, you can move up the body to the arms and hands.
3. *Tummy and chest:* These areas may be more sensitive, so be extra gentle.
4. *Face:* Babies' faces can be tense due to sucking, crying, and smiling.

5. *Back:* Massaging the back is very relaxing for babies, and some babies will fall asleep in this position.

NOTE: *Never leave babies sleeping in a facedown position.*

Effleurage: The Basic Stress-Relief Massage Stroke

A soothing Swedish massage stroke, effleurage can be used on all parts of the body to warm up and loosen muscles. Simply warm oil in your hands and use your palms to apply gentle but firm pressure as you glide your hands on the skin in the direction of the heart. This helps blood and lymph flow, is deeply relaxing, and can de-stress babies and adults very quickly!

INFANT LEG MASSAGE REMEDY

Massaging the legs is a fantastic soother and stress reliever, especially when babies start to crawl and stand up. It improves circulation and relaxes and tones baby's muscles. The soles of the feet have thousands of reflexology points that correspond to different parts of the body, and pressing on them can help relax baby's entire body.

    When you move your hands from the thigh to the ankle, it's called "Indian milking," which moves negative energy and stress from the trunk of the body toward (and out) the feet. When you begin at the ankle and stroke toward the thigh, it's called "Swedish milking," which encourages energy to move toward the heart rather than toward the extremities. They're equally comforting and beneficial. These massage terms were first introduced by Vimala Schneider McClure, the foremost authority on infant massage, who brought infant massage techniques to the United States from India in 1978.

1. *Squeezing and releasing:* Place one hand on top of the baby's upper thigh and the other hand under the thigh. Gently squeeze with both hands and re-lease the leg, as you move from the top of the thigh down to the ankle. As you work your way down the leg, switch one hand over the other, as if you were climbing a rope. Use gentle, firm pressure, maintaining as much con-sistency as possible. Keep your movements slow and smooth. Repeat two or three times. Next, do the same squeeze and release starting at the ankle and moving up toward the top of baby's thigh. Repeat two or three times.

2. *Squeezing and twisting:* Beginning at the top of the thigh, hold the baby's leg with both hands and gently squeeze and twist your hands around the leg, moving down toward the ankle.

3. *Rolling:* Place your hands on either side of baby's leg at the top of the thigh, and gently roll the leg between your hands from the thigh to the ankle (as if you're rolling a cord of dough). Rolling the muscles stimulates the baby's nerves, relaxes the muscles, and reduces stress.

4. *Feathering:* Finish the leg massage by using your fingertips to lightly stroke down the baby's entire leg from the hip to the toes. This touch has less pressure—in fact, it's barely perceptible to the baby, yet it has a profoundly soothing effect. Feathering helps integrate the legs with the trunk and provides a sense of closure for this part of the massage.

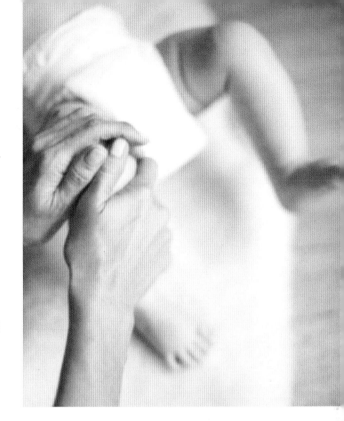

INFANT FOOT MASSAGE REMEDY

1. *Thumb-stroking soles:* Hold the foot with one hand; with your other hand use your thumb to apply gentle, firm pressure and stroke lightly along the bottom of the foot. The feet have many reflexology points that correspond to specific parts of the body. Follow the reflexology chart (p. 21) and press on areas where baby may need help. Newborns who received needle pricks on their feet while in the hospital may be sensitive in this area, so be extra gentle.

2. *Squeezing and rotating:* Squeeze and rotate each toe.

3. *Thumb-stroking top and ankle:* Thumb-stroke along the top of the foot, toward the ankle, and then stroke around the ankle.

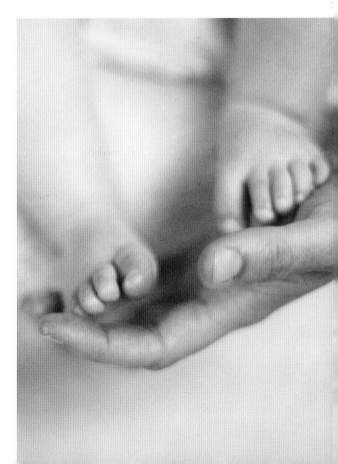

4. *Stretching and rotating:* Gently pull back on the ball of the foot and then slowly rotate the foot in one direction, then in the other.

5. *Feathering:* Use the same stroke as on the legs, but apply a bit more pressure to the feet.

INFANT ARM MASSAGE REMEDY

Massaging the arms not only helps baby relax, but it also encourages baby to open up to the world. Newborns tend to pull their arms in close to their chests when they feel vulnerable. If you try to extend their arms, you're almost guaranteed a struggle. However, when a baby finally lets go and relaxes for an arm massage, it's a sign of trust. The arms can be one of the trickiest areas to massage on a baby. Be patient—it's worth it!

TIP: *If your baby withdraws from you and pulls the arms into the chest, try taking your baby's hand in yours. Raise it slightly in the air and gently wiggle it back and forth. Babies usually respond to this and will release the tension in their arms and hands, allowing you to continue the massage. However, if your baby does not release the arm tension, simply move on to another part of the body and come back to the arms later to try again.*

1. *Squeezing and releasing:* Place one hand on top of baby's arm and the other hand under the arm. Gently squeeze and release the arm as you move from the shoulder down to the wrist. Work your way down the arm switching hand over hand. Use gentle, firm pressure, maintaining as much consistency as possible. Keep your movements slow and smooth. Repeat two or three times. Next, do the same squeeze and release starting at the wrist and moving up toward the shoulder. Repeat two or three times.

2. *Squeezing and twisting:* This stroke begins at the top of the shoulder and moves down to the wrist. Hold the baby's arm with both hands and gently squeeze and twist your hands around it, moving toward the wrist. Squeeze baby's arm firmly, so that there's some pressure, but not so tightly that you pull at the skin. With oil, your hands should just glide back and forth over the skin squeezing, twisting, and then releasing slightly, so that your hands can move down to the wrist a bit more. Do this several times.

3. *Rolling:* Place your hands on either side of baby's arm near the shoulder, and gently roll the arm between your hands from the shoulder to the

wrist (as if you were trying to roll a cord of dough). Rolling the muscles stimulates the baby's nerves, relaxes muscles, and reduces stress.

4. *Feathering:* Finish the arm massage by using your fingertips to lightly stroke down the baby's entire arm several times. This brushes out the energy through the hands.

INFANT HAND MASSAGE REMEDY

When babies are stressed they often clench their hands into tight fists. Massaging their hands can help release tension and encourage babies to relax both their hands and arms. There are also thousands of reflexology points on the hands that you can press to help soothe and comfort a baby.

1. *Thumb-stroking palms:* Use your thumbs to apply gentle, firm pressure and stroke lightly on the palm of the hand. Try to cover the entire palm.

2. *Squeezing and rotating:* Squeeze and rotate each finger.

3. *Thumb-stroking top of hand and wrist:* Stroke the top of the hand and wrist with your thumbs.

4. *Stretching and rotating:* Gently stretch the hand forward and back, and then rotate in one direction, then the other.

INFANT TUMMY MASSAGE REMEDY

Massaging your baby's belly can provide much needed relief from gas and constipation (who doesn't want that?!). If baby is fussy, just a few minutes of massaging the belly, even over clothing, can work wonders.

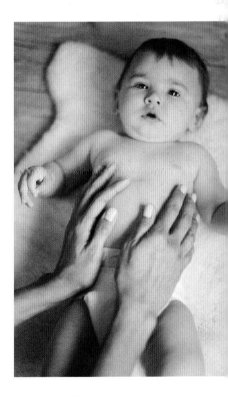

Tummy Massage Guidelines

1. Make sure the umbilical cord is completely healed before massaging the tummy.

2. When massaging in a circular motion, always massage in a *clockwise* direction. The purpose of tummy massage is to help move gas and waste matter toward the bowels, and the strokes should always follow the natural direction of the colon, which is from baby's right side to

baby's left side, which, when you're facing the baby, is from your left to your right. Stroking in a counterclockwise direction pushes things in the wrong direction and can upset your baby's delicate intestinal system.

3. *Down stroke:* With alternating hands, stroke your palms downward from the rib cage to the top of the legs. Scoop your palms down and up with gentle, but firm pressure. Repeat several times. Gas relief is on the way!

4. *Circle stroke:* Massage clockwise around the navel. Some people call this stroke the "I Love You" stroke, because the three steps of the stroke look like the letters "I" and "L" and "U." I like to do each of the strokes several times, and then put the "I Love You" sequence together as the circle stroke.

"I": With your *right* hand, stroke an "I." Place your hand just below baby's rib cage on baby's left side (your right). Stroke straight down to the bottom of the belly.

"L": With your *left* hand, stroke an upside-down "L." Place your hand just below baby's right rib cage (your left), move your hand horizontally to your right to just below baby's left rib cage, and then straight down, to the lower left side of baby's belly.

"U": With your *right* hand stroke an upside-down "U" and complete the "I love you." Place your hand on the lower belly on baby's right side (your left), move up toward the rib cage, then stroke your hand horizontally to baby's left side (your right), and then straight down. With this final "U" stroke you trace over where you did the "I" and "L" strokes.

"I love you": Massage a complete circle with your hands moving clockwise over the entire "I love you" and continuing under the belly button. Use both hands; just alternate right hand over left hand, moving in a continuous circle. Keep your pressure light.

5. *Thumb stroke:* Place thumbs together on baby's belly, just below the rib cage, and gently push outward moving your thumbs out to the sides of baby's body. Move down an inch and repeat until below the belly button. Repeat several times. If your baby has gas, this stroke may cause fussiness. If you can continue the massage, you'll help move the gas through his system more quickly.

6. *Paddling:* Hold both of baby's legs together with one hand at the ankles. Use your other hand to make paddling strokes on your baby's tummy (as

if you're scooping sand toward yourself). You'll find that this relaxes the tummy greatly.

7. *Tummy stretch:* To complete the tummy massage, bring your baby's legs in toward to the chest (with knees bent), then release. This helps digestion, pushes gas out of the body, and integrates the rest of the body.

WARNING: *It's not unusual to have babies relieve themselves during or after a tummy massage. Be prepared to clean up the mess or change a diaper!*

INFANT CHEST MASSAGE REMEDY

Massaging the chest can help relieve congestion and help your baby's heart and lungs. It helps to relax babies who often keep their arms closed protectively over their chests. Babies love this and respond by relaxing their arms, so that their chest opens up to you.

1. *Heart stroke:* Place both hands together on the center of baby's chest. Gently stroke your hands from the center of the chest up to the collarbone, and then outward to the sides, bringing them back together in a heart-shaped motion at the center. Do this several times, massaging hearts across your baby's chest.

2. *Butterfly stroke:* Place your hands on each side of baby, at the bottom of the rib cage. Beginning with your right hand, stroke diagonally across the chest toward baby's right shoulder, and stroke back down across the chest, following the same line that you just made. Your left hand follows this same movement but moves diagonally toward baby's left shoulder and back down. Continue to crisscross over the chest, alternating hands, several times.

AROMATHERAPY TO RELIEVE CONGESTION

4 drops fir needle or cypress oil
2 drops lavender oil
2 ounces unscented natural oil

Use this blend of aromatherapy essential oils to help relieve your baby's chest or sinus congestion due to a cold or allergies. After combining the oils, place a few drops on the palm of one hand, then rub your hands together. Massaging the chest with this soothing aromatherapy blend will help your baby breathe easier.

INFANT FACE MASSAGE REMEDY

Many babies, particularly during the first three months, carry stress in their face from crying, sucking, teething, and interacting with the world. Massaging your baby's face is a great way to relieve this tension, make eye contact, and really bond with your baby.

TIP: *Some babies may cry if hands are placed on their face too quickly, which causes a startle reflex. To prevent this, begin the face massage by slowly placing your hands on baby's cheeks. Hold them here for a few seconds, so the baby can feel the warmth of your hands. This can relax your baby, so he or she is open to a face massage.*

1. *Forehead:* Place your thumbs on the center of the forehead and slowly slide them outward to the hairline. Repeat several times to cover the entire forehead.

2. *Nose, cheeks, and jaw:* Place the tips of the index and middle fingers on either side of the nose. Stroke outward to the temples, then repeat, each time moving your fingertips down the cheeks to the chin and jawline.

3. *Eyes:* With your middle fingers, slowly trace circles around baby's eyes several times. Then stroke the eyebrows from the inside edge to the outside edge.

4. *Head:* Use the palms of both hands to stroke baby's head from front to crown.

INFANT BACK MASSAGE REMEDY

A back massage is extremely relaxing for babies who have been trying to lift their heads and crawl.

WARNING: *When placed facedown during massage, baby is likely to fall asleep quickly. Never leave a sleeping baby in the facedown position after a massage. If baby falls asleep, gently turn baby onto the back. You can continue to massage and lull baby into a deeper sleep or stop massaging. When a baby falls asleep, I usually stop massaging and keep my hands still on the back for 15 to 20 seconds, when I'm sure baby is fully asleep. Then I very slowly remove my hands, so baby doesn't feel an abrupt movement.*

1. *Position:* Turn your baby on his or her stomach horizontally in front of you. Babies generally turn their heads to face you in this position.

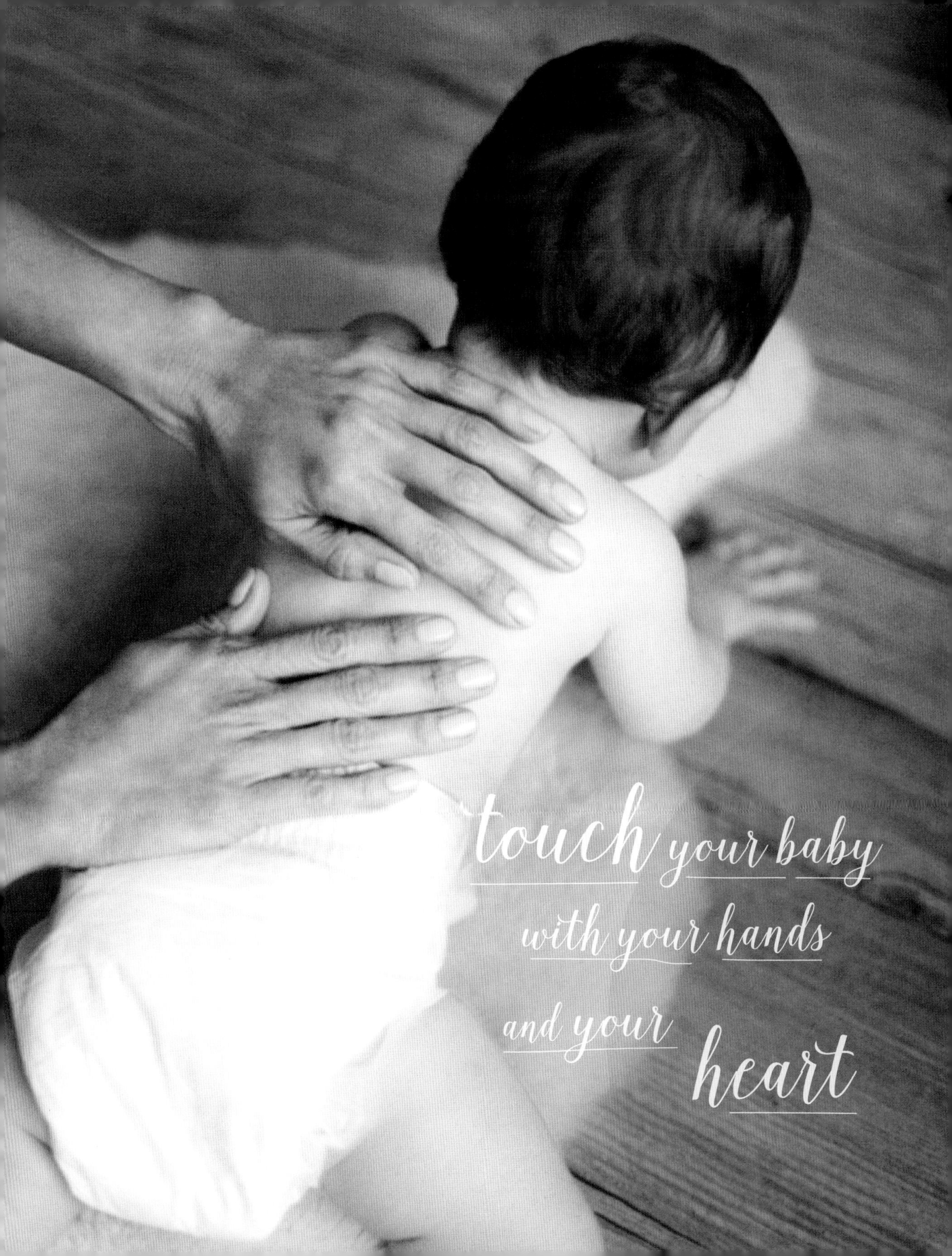

touch your baby
with your hands
and your
heart

2. *Down stroke:* Place one hand on baby's buttocks and with the other hand stroke down the back several times, from the shoulder to the buttocks. Try to cover baby's entire back.

3. *Across the back:* Place your hands on the middle of baby's back, perpendicular to the spine, and glide them back and forth in opposite directions from one side to the other. Try to cover the entire back.

4. *Small circles:* Make small circles all over the back with the palms of your hands, moving them from one side of the spine to the other.

5. *Cat stroke:* With the pads of your fingertips, stroke down the back several times from the neck to the buttocks. Make each stroke lighter, until it turns into the feather touch you've already used.

Fussy Baby Remedies

COLIC-RELIEF MASSAGE REMEDY

Nothing is more distressing to a parent than an inconsolable newborn who won't stop crying. Massaging your baby's belly can significantly reduce the amount of time spent crying by helping to relieve gas and constipation, so that your baby's system functions better. It may take a few days for your baby to respond, but have patience, continue to massage regularly, and you'll both benefit.

Some babies get colic. Colic is defined by doctors as "inconsolable crying that occurs during a baby's first three months, that lasts at least three hours a day, three days a week, and continues for three weeks." In addition to excessive crying, there's also fussiness, sensitivity, and wakefulness. (It's *hell*! I know.) According to the American Academy of Pediatrics, approximately one in five infants, usually between the ages of two and four weeks, develop colic, which ends when they're three to five months.[13] In the words of one physician, "You know your baby has colic when you have the irresistible urge to get him his own apartment."

Doctors don't know the exact cause of colic, but possible reasons are an immature gastrointestinal system and central nervous system, and the baby's temperament (which is quite distressing to parents!). The good news is that, as the nervous system matures at around three to six months, colicky babies usually calm down.

TIP: *Each technique can be done with or without baby's clothes on. Do each step several times.*

1. *Tummy rocking:* Lay your baby on the back. Facing your baby, hold the ankles and gently push the knees together toward the belly; then stretch the legs out straight. When you bring baby's legs inward, gently rock the legs from side to side, so that baby releases and relaxes the knees. When you straighten baby's legs, gently rock the hips, so that baby relaxes and extends the legs.

2. *Bicycling:* Slowly bend and stretch each leg in bicycling motion. Do this slowly, so that each leg can straighten all the way. Babies usually enjoy this.

3. *Leg cross:* Cross the legs at the belly and gently press them in toward the belly. This should help baby release some gas. Hold for a few seconds and then straighten them. Then reverse legs, with the other leg crossed in front.

4. *Paddling:* Place the palms of your hands horizontally on baby's belly, just below the rib cage. Alternating hands, glide your palms down toward the legs using a scooping motion. Apply gentle, firm pressure.

5. *Tummy massage:* Do any or all of the Infant Tummy Massage Remedy techniques.

AROMATHERAPY FOR COLICKY BABIES

5 drops lavender oil
3 drops of Roman chamomile oil
3 drops sweet orange oil
2 ounces unscented oil

Combine these oils and apply a few drops to the palm of one hand. Rub your hands together and then do the remedies for fussy babies. The calming scent will relax baby and ease colic.

Research published in the *International Journal of Nursing Practice* showed that "the use of aromatherapy massage using lavender oil was found to be effective in reducing the symptoms of colic."[14]

INFANT CALMING THERAPEUTIC-TOUCH REMEDY

There may be times when babies are so irritable that massage is not an option. Also, there are babies who are stimulated by massage, which is not what you want to do when trying to encourage sleep. This soothing therapeutic-touch remedy is a gentle and safe way to soothe fussy babies and help them sleep. The aromatherapy blend for colic is also very effective to use here.

Therapeutic touch is a gentle, noninvasive therapy that decreases stress, anxiety, and pain in adults and children by balancing the flow of energy in the body. In a study at Texas Tech University, infants who were treated with therapeutic touch responded with "reduced heart and respiratory rates, enhanced ability to rest, improved coordination in sucking, swallowing, and breathing, and a greater ability to engage with the environment."[15]

I. *Burrito swaddling* (also referred to as "containing" in therapeutic touch): Lay a blanket in a diamond shape and fold the top corner down to form a triangle. Place baby on top and pull one side of blanket across baby's chest and tuck under the opposite arm. Fold the bottom of blanket over the feet and tuck it behind baby's shoulder. Pull the remaining side of blanket across the baby's chest and tuck it underneath. Your baby is now properly swaddled into a cozy burrito.

2. *Hand smoothing:* Sit in a comfortable position and hold your baby close in your arms (as if you were breastfeeding). Take your free hand and place it on the back of baby's head, allowing the weight of the head to relax into your hand. Keep your hand still and just hold this position for several minutes. The warmth of your hand will calm baby. Then, with your baby's head supported in the crook of your arm, use the palm of your hand to gently stroke baby's head from front to back. Do this several times very slowly.

Toddlers and Tikes

Mothers hold their children's hands for a short while, but their hearts forever.
—ANONYMOUS

As babies grow and their needs change, daily touch is often one of the first things that parents overlook. But regular massage shouldn't end when babies become toddlers! Although toddlers and tikes (twelve and under) may not need to be held, rocked, cared for, and watched over 24/7 anymore, they still *need* touch as much, if not more, than when they were babies! With digital devices and screens vying for their attention, kids needs time and space to connect with you. Daily touch therapy can fill that need. Although the baby massage remedies can still be used on older children, the touch remedies in

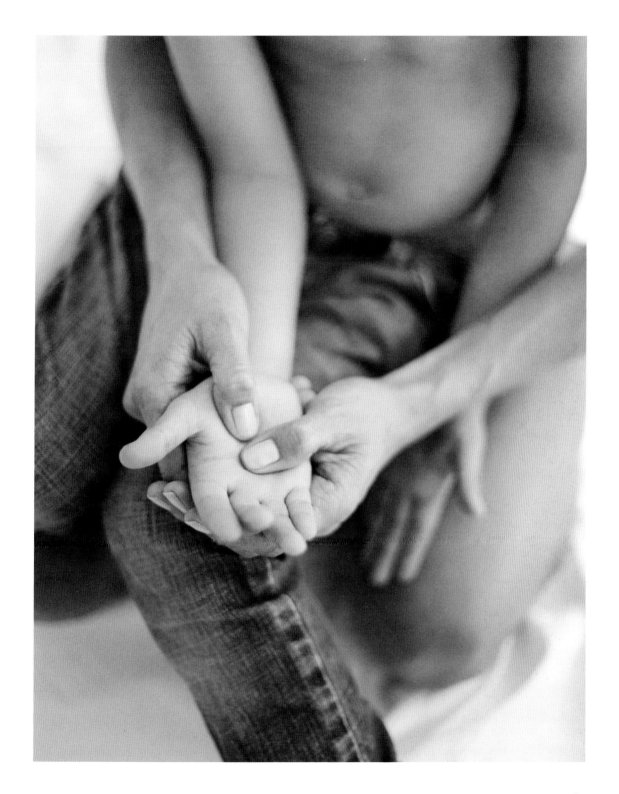

this chapter are modified techniques to accommodate the unique physical, emotional and psychological needs of kids at each stage of growth and development.

Toddlers' lives can be very frustrating, because they want to do more than their skills allow. As they naturally strive to literally and figuratively move away from their parents, their need for emotional and physical connection grows. While demanding their autonomy ("No!" is their favorite word), toddlers still need parents' help and guidance, especially when it comes to winding down and learning how to relax. Slowing down and de-stressing is an important lesson at this age. Encouraging children to be still and tune into the soothing sensations of touch teaches them how to let go of stress, which will help them throughout their life.

Even if touch therapy at this age consists of just a 5-minute quickie that happens when you can get your child to stay still, using touch on children regularly can help parents become sensitive caretakers attuned to their children's needs. It can help children sleep better and feel more confident and relaxed. It can also help build an intimate relationship based on trust and restore harmony after a difficult day with a demanding toddler or school-age child. Touch may have to be on their terms, but it will benefit both of you in the end.

When parents respond to their child's needs with compassion and sensitivity, the child will grow up to respect and trust their positive authority. Another bonus is that parents often find their children are less aggressive toward one another and that the home becomes more peaceful after massage is introduced. According to Shay Beider, founder and executive director of Integrative Touch for Kids, "The essence of massage for children is providing safe and loving touch that encourages a positive experience in the body and that nurtures healthy relationships."[16]

Effects of Massage on Children

All the benefits of baby massage mentioned earlier apply to young children as well (enhancing communication, relaxing and soothing the nervous system, helping with sleep, etc.). In addition, clinical studies at the University of Miami's Touch Research Institute prove that massage helps children with a number of special conditions, including:

- *Anxiety:* A study that compared children who were massaged to a control group of children who viewed relaxing videotapes showed that the massaged children were "less depressed and anxious and had lower saliva cortisol levels after the massage. In addition, nighttime sleep increased over the study period and urinary cortisol and norepinephrine levels decreased."[17]

- *Autism:* Massage therapy early in life has repeatedly been shown to be an effective, low-cost therapeutic approach in improving the cognitive, social, and emotional symptoms of autism. Researchers found that children who were massaged "exhibited less stereotypic (autistic) behavior and showed more on-task and social relatedness behavior during play observations at school, and they experienced fewer sleep problems at home" than those who were not massaged. In this study, parents who were trained by a massage therapist massaged their children for 15 minutes before bedtime every night for one month.[18]

- *Asthma:* Children were given 20 minutes of massage by their parents before bedtime each night for thirty days, and were compared to a control group who received relaxation therapy. The children who received massage therapy showed an immediate decrease in behavioral anxiety and cortisol levels after massage as well as improved pulmonary function.[19]

- *ADHD:* Two studies report that regular massage therapy can be an effective treatment for kids with ADHD. One study on adolescent boys, who received ten 15-minute daily massages, showed they were more focused in their schoolwork, and they fidgeted less. In addition, the boys rated themselves as happier than those who participated in another relaxation-therapy program. Another study involved kids aged seven to eighteen (20 percent were girls). Each subject received a 20-minute massage twice a week. They all showed immediate improvement in their moods and longer-term behavioral improvement in the classroom. They also reported feeling happier and their teachers found them to be more attentive.[20]

- *Cerebral palsy:* Twenty young children with cerebral palsy received 30 minutes of massage or reading twice weekly for twelve weeks. The children receiving massage therapy showed fewer physical symptoms including "reduced spasticity, less rigid muscle tone overall and in the arms, and improved fine and gross motor functioning." In addition, the massage group showed more positive facial expressions and less limb activity during face-to-face play interactions.[21]

- *Down syndrome:* In a study, high-functioning young Down syndrome children were randomly assigned to receive two 30-minute massage therapy or reading sessions per week for two months. Children in the massage group revealed greater gains in fine and gross motor functioning when compared with the children in the reading control group.[22]

Handling Children with Special Needs

Parents should be aware that many children with special needs, especially those diagnosed on the autism spectrum and those with sensory differences, can have anxiety about touch as well as vulnerability to sensory overload; they may have tactile hypersensitivities or have interpreted previous touch as painful or confusing. According to Tina Allen, founder of the leading children's health and nurturing touch organization, Liddle Kidz Foundation: "Parents should move cautiously (keep transitions slow) and respect the child's cues. Take time to recognize a child's likes and dislikes associated with types of touch, textures, sensory considerations and type of lubricant (oil/lotion). Permission is imperative and parents should recognize their children might not always provide direct eye-to-eye contact or a verbal 'Yes.'"[23] Consult your physician if you have concerns.

FAQs

How is massage for kids different from massage for adults?

Kids respond differently to massage than adults, typically becoming more actively engaged and interested in what you're doing and why. Physiologically, kids' nervous systems are more delicate than adults; they have more touch receptors per square inch than adults and their skin is more porous and, therefore, more sensitive than adults'. As a result, touch-therapy techniques for kids require more open communication, lighter pressure, and sometimes imagination to make toddlers more receptive to it.[24]

How can I make massage more fun for a toddler?

1. *Tell a story:* Place your hands on your child's back and tell a story while drawing images of what's happening on the back. For example, I like to tell a story about a boat with a big sail, which I outline with my fingers. Then I make slow circular movements to portray a calm sea with small waves and, later, quicker larger circles to portray a storm with big waves. You can draw small fish, big whales, starfish, raindrops, whatever you want, all the while making up a story to go along with what your fingers are drawing. This really keeps little ones engaged!

2. *Play "Guess the Letter/Number":* This game is fun for kids who are learning the alphabet and numbers. Trace a letter or number on your child's back and ask your child to guess what it is. Later, you can spell words to practice spelling skills.

How can I help my child feel comfortable with massage?

By building trust. You can do that by always asking permission before giving a massage. If the answer is no, respect that. Learning that it's okay to say no to unwelcome touch is a very important message to give children. It teaches them about boundaries. By respecting your child's boundaries you can help him or her feel safe, which builds trust. Soon enough your child will realize that massage is something that feels good and will be asking for one regularly! Help your child recognize his or her preferences and responses to touch. For example, ask, "How does that feel?" and "What part of your body do you like massaged the most?"

Tips to Keep in Mind

- Be mindful of your child's attention span.
- Continue to communicate during the massage.
- Be aware of subtle changes in your child's behavior. The child may become quiet or agitated if feeling uncomfortable and may not be able to express this in words.

Effleurage: The Basic Stress-Relief Massage Stroke

Effleurage, a soothing Swedish massage stroke, can be used on all parts of the body to warm up and loosen muscles. Using your palms to apply gentle, firm pressure as you glide your hands in the direction of the heart helps blood and lymph flow and is deeply relaxing. Practicing it on the back is helpful and a very soothing way to begin the massage.

TRANQUILITY MASSAGE REMEDY FOR TODDLERS

Toddlers are often interested in exploring their environment and enjoy massage that is active and engaging. Toddlers who are constantly on the go benefit tremendously from soothing massage strokes that relax their muscles and calm their minds after a busy day.

1. *Position:* Lay a towel on a bed or couch, and have the child lie flat on the tummy. In this prone position, kids tend to calm down and relax. You can either massage over clothes with no oil or, depending on how comfortable the child is, massage using oil with clothes off. Sometimes kids feel more comfortable just removing their shirt for a back massage. Always ask the child what feels comfortable.

2. *Back:* Position yourself on one side, and place the palms of your hands on either side of the spine at the lower back. (If you're using oil, warm some oil in your hands.) Apply some pressure and slowly bring your hands up the back to the base of the neck, out to the edge of each shoulder, and then back down the back. Tell the child to take a deep breath and close the eyes. Repeat several times. Ask the child how it feels.

3. *Arms:* After several minutes stroking the back, glide your hands up to the shoulders and then bring them down each arm, all the way to the hands. When you get to the hands, massage all the way to the ends of the child's fingertips. Do this several times, trying to touch the whole arm.

4. *Legs:* To transition down to the legs, do a few back effleurages and then glide your hands over the buttocks and down the legs to the feet. You will have to move down closer to the child's feet. Glide your hands from the soles of the feet, up the back of the legs to just below the buttocks, and back down.

5. *Feet:* I like to end by placing the palms of both hands on the soles of the feet, and slowly stroking from the heel to the toes several times.

NEW WALKERS MASSAGE REMEDY

Toddlers who are just getting comfortable using their legs to stand and walk often have tired muscles that need relaxing. This touch remedy improves the circulation in their legs and de-stresses their entire lower body.

1. *Position:* Have the child lie on the back. You can do this remedy pants off with oil or on top of clothing with no oil.

2. *Effleurage and squeeze:* Place your hands on one ankle and apply light pressure as you effleurage up the leg to the top of the thigh and back down. Next, as you glide your hands up and down the leg, stop every 3 inches and give the leg a tender squeeze. Repeat these two alternating strokes three times on each leg.

3. *Ringing:* Place the palms of your hands horizontally on one leg and alternate gliding your hands in a back-and-forth motion across the leg, from side to side, moving upward slowly from the ankle to the top of the thigh, and back down. As you bring your palms up, gently lift the muscle. Do this three times on each leg.

4. *Effleurage, both legs together:* Place one hand on each leg and apply gentle pressure as you effleurage up the legs and back down. As you move up the legs apply slightly more pressure to encourage the blood flow toward the heart. As you bring your hands down, lighten the pressure. Do this several times.

5. *Backs of the legs:* Have the child turn over and repeat these same steps on the backs of the legs.

Remedies for High-Energy 'Spirited' Children

"SPIRITED CHILD" TOUCH REMEDY

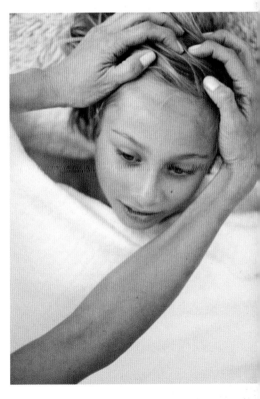

Parents of high-energy children know that getting them to slow down for even just a few minutes can be quite challenging. This technique, which is helpful for autism, Asperger's, and ADHD, is a quick way to cut out external stimuli and help your child to turn inward, so he or she can tune into the soothing sensations of a head massage.

1. *Burrito wrap:* Find a cozy blanket and lay it out on the floor. Fold the top corner of the blanket down and have the child lie in the middle with the head on the folded part. Bring one side of the blanket over and tuck it under the child. Fold the bottom up. Wrap the remaining side over and around the child. The child should feel cozy and secure in this wrap, which holds the limbs still, but not too tight. You can also cover the child in another blanket for added weight. Occupational

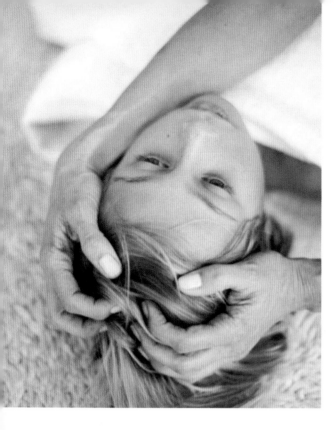

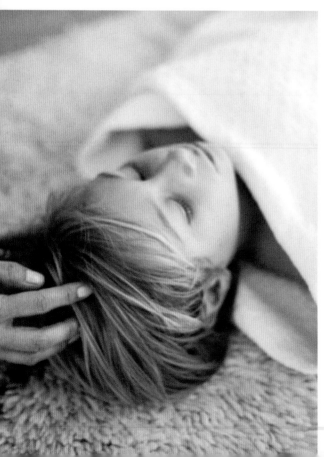

therapists sometimes use this technique of weighted blankets for children with sensory-processing disorders. It helps to calm them, improves their attention and focusing ability, decreases sensory-seeking behaviors, and has an organizing effect on the central nervous system.

2. *Acupressure head massage:* Sit near the child's head and place your fingertips on the top of the head, in the middle close to the forehead. Ask the child to close eyes, be quiet, and think about what he or she is feeling on the head. Apply a little pressure with your fingers and make small circles very slowly, count to 5, then move your fingertips an inch out toward the ears. Repeat, so that you cover the entire scalp.

3. *"Calming" point:* Place the three middle fingers of both hands on the crown of the head and hold there for 10 to 15 seconds. To find the exact "calming" point, follow a line from the back of both ears to the top of the head. Feel for a slight hollow toward the back of the top of the head. This is called the "Hundred Meetings" point in traditional Chinese medicine, and applying gentle pressure here is helpful for mental concentration, improving memory, and headaches.

Touchy Tweens and Teens

Adolescence is a period of rapid changes. Between the ages of twelve and seventeen, a parent ages as much as twenty years.

—Anonymous

Why Touch Is So Needed During Adolescence

When kids hit the tween/teen years, which are those lovely years frequently characterized by hormone-fueled bouts of moodiness, rudeness, self-consciousness, risk taking, sleeping until noon, and other obnoxious behavior, parents often take cover. Walking on eggshells around their teenager, not only are they disturbed by their child's new demeanor; they're afraid of doing or saying something that might set off even worse behavior. For most parents, even those who used touch therapy during their child's growing years, this is often the beginning of the end of touching their children.

Unfortunately, this comes at a time when children need their parents' touch as much as ever, since adolescents are in the midst of tremendous physical and emotional developmental changes that are out of their control. They still need the comfort of touch from people they trust. This is also an important time for parents to extend their teaching about boundaries, respect, and unwelcome touch, underscoring that there are different types of touch, some sexual and many nonsexual, and how to distinguish between the two. Adolescents must learn about boundaries, that their body is their own, and that they can always say no to any touch that makes them uncomfortable.

What's most frustrating during this stage is that, although adolescents may still want and need reassuring, comforting touch, they often outwardly avoid their parents' touch in an effort to "break free" and appear more independent and mature. They're caught in the phase when they're "too old" to seek comfort from cuddling, yet "too young" to find comfort from deeper, sexual adult relationships. Ironically, as an adolescent's need for touch increases during this time, many parents avoid touching their children when they approach puberty due to their own discomfort. It's a *lose-lose* situation for both parent and child.

In addition, "touch avoidance" is required at some schools across the country that have policies prohibiting hugging, hand-holding, and other forms of affection between students and between students and teachers.[25] In 2012, Tennessee senators actually passed legislation, labeled the "No Holding Hands Bill" by critics, that bans "gateway sexual activity." Legislators claimed that the bill would prevent "unsuitable interactions" between students, but the bill defines "gateway sexual activity" so vaguely that it could include pretty much anything teenagers do that involves touch.[26] At an age when holding hands and hugging are ways for kids to bridge the gap between child and adult behavior, this type of policy can be detrimental to adolescents, who should be learning how to navigate personal interactions and build healthy relationships.

As a mother of a tween, I can honestly say that touch therapy (a back massage before bed, in particular) is my way of holding on to a connection with my eldest son, who is on the verge of abandoning boyhood and about to enter adolescence. He still welcomes my cuddles, and for that I am grateful. My two other little guys are always up for a snuggle, a minimassage, and some alone time with mom. The touch-therapy remedies that follow work for me, and I know they'll work for you.

The Benefits

Every parent knows how tough the tween/teen years can be. More and more research is demonstrating that one of the most critical factors in ensuring the well-being of today's adolescents is parent involvement. My noninvasive touch remedies can help you get involved and stay in touch with your child as well as:

- Communicate and connect with a child who's changing in front of your eyes
- Encourage an uncommunicative teen to relax and open up
- Provide real quality time
- Teach children how to calm down, bring awareness to what's inside of them, and tap into their own internal compass
- Strengthen the parent-child bond, which aids in substance abuse prevention, violence prevention, and positive character development

The Remedies

5-MINUTE INTERLOCKING HAND REFLEXOLOGY REMEDY

Your child may not be comfortable holding hands with you while walking down the street, but I'm pretty sure he or she will gladly give them to you for this all-over anxiety soother. The face-to-face position encourages an intimate connection. It's a great remedy to relax your child, so that he or she can naturally open up and communicate with you. Two and a half minutes for each hand is all you need!

1. Sit facing each other or, if on a couch, angled toward each other, and interlock the fingers of both of your hands with one of the child's hands so that the palm opens up. It helps to place a pillow under your hands for support.

2. Keep your hands interlocked and place your thumbs in the center of the palm, which is the reflex area to the solar plexus (the "nerve center of the body"). Apply firm pressure and make small circles with your thumb in one direction several times, and then in the other direction. This can relax the entire body.

3. Alternately, rub each thumb outward from the center of the palm toward the outer edges of the palm. Try to cover the entire palm.

4. Repeat on the other hand.

5. Holding one hand in yours for support, use your other hand to rub each finger between your thumb and index finger, from the base of the finger to the fingertips.

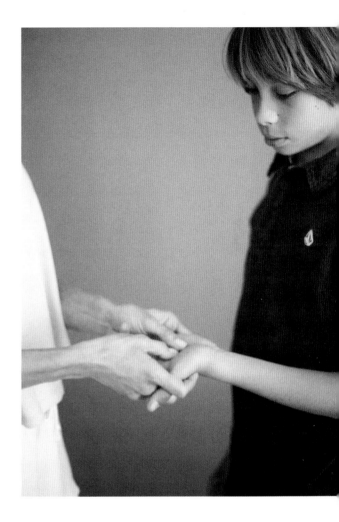

HOMEWORK HELPER
CRANIAL-SACRAL REMEDY

Most kids need some help transitioning from afterschool activities into "homework mode." This relaxing yet energizing technique will help refocus your child's attention and boost energy, so your child is ready to tackle homework.

1. Stand behind your child, who is sitting in a chair. With the child's eyes closed, place your hands over the ears for 10 seconds. This shuts out external stimulation and quickly helps the child to turn inward.

2. Place your fingertips on the top of the head and slowly make small circles all over to invigorate the scalp. Do this for 2 to 3 minutes.

3. Place your fingertips on the top of the head, on either side of the center part. Apply light pressure beginning with your pinkie, then the next finger, and the next, until all fingers have applied pressure—almost as if you're playing the piano on the head. Do this several times and then hold for 5 seconds. Repeat, and then move your hands farther back, following the center part line at the back of the head. This light, gentle pressure and slight rocking motion allows the skull to relax. It's a cranial-sacral technique that encourages the cranial-sacral fluid to move more freely in the brain and through the spine.

4. Place your fingertips just under the ridge at the back of the head and apply gentle, firm pressure upward. Ask the child to slowly tilt the head backward, allowing the weight of the head to fall into your hands.

RELAXING INCENTIVE REFLEXOLOGY REMEDY

All parents need something they can use to bribe a teenager! This remedy is extremely soothing, and your teen will love it so much that you can use it as an incentive to get him or her to do whatever you want. Even though it's a foot massage, it can effectively relax the entire body.

1. Have the child lie on the back on a couch or bed and position yourself comfortably at the feet. With socks either on or off, take one foot in your hands and place your thumbs on the sole of the foot (in the middle of the foot). This is the reflex area to the solar plexus, the nerve center of the body, and pressing directly on this point can bring instant stress relief. Make small circles with your thumbs here for 30 seconds.

2. Place your thumbs on the heel, closer to the inner edge of the foot. Apply firm pressure, and alternately rub one thumb and then the other along the inner edge of the foot, which is the reflex area to the back, as you slowly move your hands up toward the big toe. This can relax the entire spine and neck.

3. When you reach the big toe, apply pressure to the big toe by rolling it between your thumb and fingers. This stimulates the reflex area to the brain, located on both big toes in the fleshy part behind the nail. This can calm the mind and soothe anxiety. Press firmly on the pad of the big toe for 10 seconds, and then make small circles with your thumb.

4. Take the foot in both hands and gently roll it between your palms.

5. Repeat on the other foot.

College Kids

Education is the best provision for life's journey.
—ARISTOTLE

Let's face it. College students are not known for making self-care a priority. (I know I didn't!) At the ripe old age of eighteen or nineteen, they're faced, often for the first time in their lives, with full responsibility for taking care of themselves while also managing the pressures of academics, social life, and choosing a major and career path. With the addition of health, family, or relationship issues, it's easy for college students to lose their balance and feel overwhelmed, exhausted, and stressed-out. And when that happens, self-care is the first thing to go!

The touch remedies in this section are so simple that parents can easily give their college kids an education on self-care and how to foster a healthy lifestyle, which is extremely important in this day and age. Teaching college-age kids how to use these basic touch-remedy tools to stay calm and healthy gives them a head start to be successful in college and for the rest of their lives.

Conquer College Stress

According to the American College Health Association, stress is still the number one obstacle to academic performance. Academic stress is a huge and growing problem among college students—28 percent of the students reported that their teachers were stressed, 39 percent reported their parents were stressed, and 35 percent reported that they themselves were stressed "often" or "very often."[27] So it makes sense that this period of young adulthood is actually the perfect time to learn self-care techniques that can be used forever to help reduce stress and function better. Learning when it's time to take a break, slow down, and engage in thoughtful self-nurturing is a lesson that's as important as any academic class! Above all, it's essential that college kids learn to recognize signs of distress in themselves and then have effective coping strategies to help them deal with stress so they can lead a healthier lifestyle.

When I was a freshman at Columbia University, I was introduced to touch therapy for the very first time at a self-acupressure workshop my friend dragged me to. I can't remember the friend's name, but the techniques I learned have become part of my own daily wellness routine for de-stressing. During college, self-acupressure helped me boost my immune system and suppress anxiety that arose all too often during class discussions and public-speaking presentations. Later, I learned to use a lymphatic massage technique to help energize myself on sleepy mornings and anytime I needed a boost.

Here are my favorite touch remedies to help manage stress effectively while in college. They're quick and easy and can be done alone (no partner needed!). So the next time coursework is piling up, all-nighters are happening, and college kids think they can't afford to take a break, they'll realize that they can't afford not to—and they'll be able to use a touch remedy to reduce their stress and improve their physical and mental health. Parents everywhere can now breathe a sigh of relief!

ENERGIZING WAKE-UP LYMPHATIC MASSAGE REMEDY

College kids are notorious for pulling all-nighters and burning the candle at both ends (late parties and 8:00 A.M. classes are *not* compatible!). This lymphatic self-massage technique will help energize your college kid first thing in the morning and any time a little power boost is needed.

Lymphatic massage is a type of gentle massage that encourages the natural drainage of the lymph fluid from the tissues of the body. You use a light pressure and rhythmic circular movements to stimulate lymph flow. By improving the circulation of blood and lymph fluids, you can help get rid of toxins, reenergize yourself, and look and feel better.

1. This can be done with or without clothes on, with your hands or with a brush (dry brushing). I like to do it before a shower or bath. Try to do it every day for maximum benefit.

2. With the palm of your hand, make small, quick circular movements going up your arms from wrist to shoulder for about 15 seconds.

3. Next, sweep up the arm, from wrist to shoulder, applying firm pressure with your palm or brush. Repeat on the other arm.

4. Continue the sweeping strokes all over the body. Begin at your feet and work your way up the body. When you get to the top of your chest,

change the direction of your strokes so that you brush down from your shoulders to your heart.

NOTE: *Always massage toward the heart.*

ACUPRESSURE AND REFLEXOLOGY REMEDY FOR STUDENT ANXIETY

College is stressful, especially when you have to perform on exams and speak in front of your classmates. Public speaking is actually the number-one fear in America. (Death is, somehow, a distant second.) And if you're being graded on your public speaking, that's a double whammy! Self-acupressure is something you can use whenever you feel stressed-out or anxious and need to calm down quickly, so you can actually think straight, focus on your exams, or get your words out. Acupressure works by tapping into your body's energy meridian system to restore balance and natural harmony. You can do it discreetly anywhere, anytime.

1. *Acupressure:* Begin by cupping your forehead in your palm and taking five deep breaths. Then take your middle and index fingers and place them on your temples, closer to the outside corners of your eyes. Apply firm pressure and then make small circles. These acupressure points are known as the "Triple Warmer" neurovasculars in acupressure. By stimulating these two points you can restore blood flow to the brain and calm your mind.

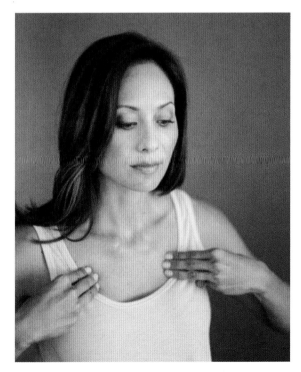

2. *Acupressure:* Use your fingertips to apply pressure on either side of your outer upper chest, 3 finger-widths below the collarbone on each side. Pressing on these acupressure points, known as "Letting Go" (LU1), can help you let go of stress, anxiety, and grief. Hold your fingers here for 15 seconds, inhaling deeply and exhaling slowly.

Letting Go Points

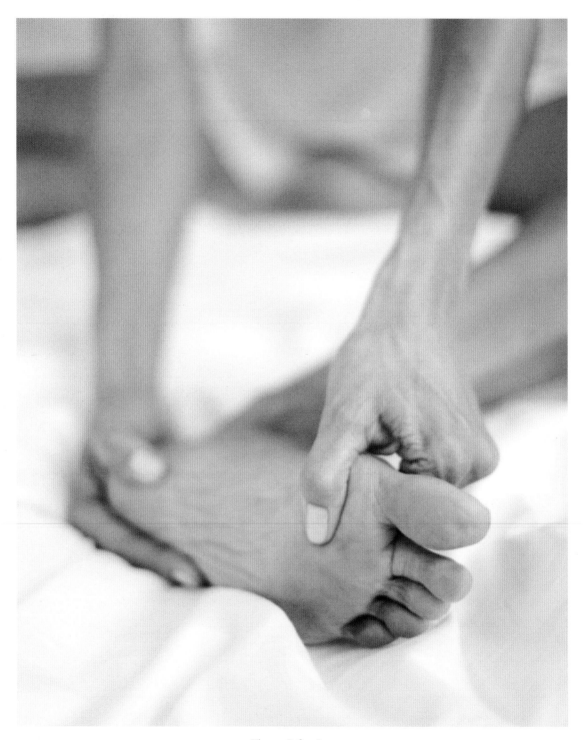

Thymus Reflex Area

3. *Reflexology:* Press the thumb of one hand into the center of the palm of the other hand. Hold for 5 to 10 seconds, then make small circles in one direction and then in the other. This stimulates the reflex area to the solar plexus, the nerve switchboard of the body, which is located in the center of the chest. Pressing here can relax your entire body.

AROMATHERAPY FOR ANXIETY

3 drops lavender oil
2 drops bergamot oil
1 drop sandalwood oil
2 ounces unscented natural oil

Before doing the remedies, rub a few drops of this aromatherapy blend between your fingertips and take a few deep inhalations of this relaxing scent.

Strengthen the Immune System

College dormitories are a breeding ground for germs. Combine that with an already weakened immune system due to an unhealthy diet, late nights, and excessive partying (I didn't do that, of course!), and you've got a recipe for sickness. Reflexology is a self-care practice that everyone can use to boost their immune system, so they can fend off all the germy dorm viruses and stay healthy.

IMMUNITY-BOOSTING REFLEXOLOGY REMEDY

1. *Thymus reflex area:* Use your thumbs to press on the inside edge of the foot, about ½ inch below the big toe. Apply firm pressure and make small circles in one direction and then the other. Stimulating this area can boost your immune system and invigorate your body.

2. *Spleen reflex area:* Move your thumbs to the outside edge of the foot and press on the sole about 1 inch below the halfway line between the heel and the toes. Stimulating this area can effective open up channels of healing energy. Again, make small circles.

3. *Brain reflex area:* Take your big toe between your thumb and index finger and apply pressure as you gently roll the big toe between your fingers. Stimulating the reflex area strengthens the immune system.

4. Repeat on the other foot.

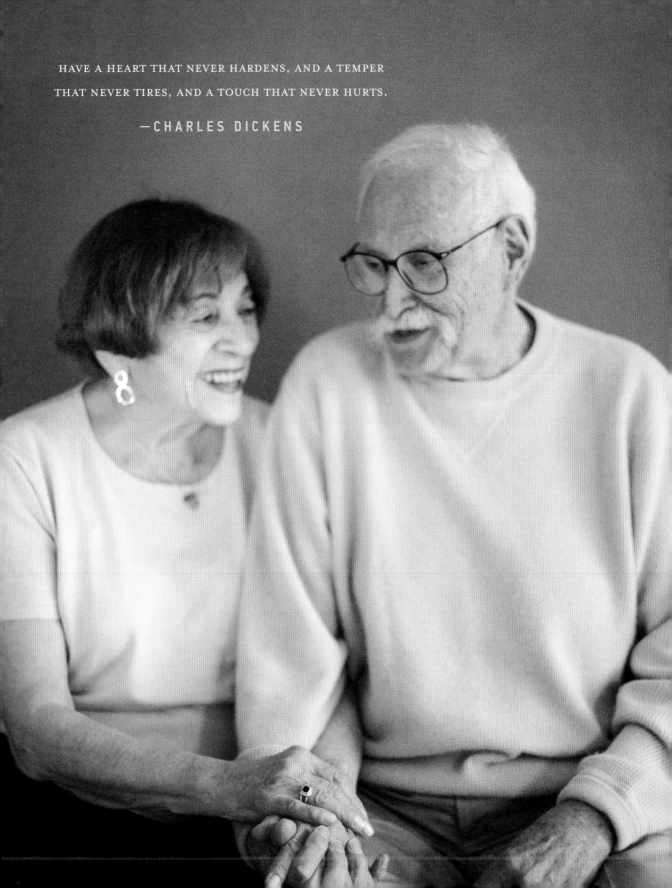

HAVE A HEART THAT NEVER HARDENS, AND A TEMPER
THAT NEVER TIRES, AND A TOUCH THAT NEVER HURTS.

—CHARLES DICKENS

CHAPTER EIGHT

Caring for the Elderly

A Labor of Love

Let's face it. Getting older is no walk in the park. Even if, as the media says, sixty is the new forty and eighty is the new sixty, in reality aging well is much more than "just a state of mind." It means having to deal with a real decline in physical function that can be challenging for anyone. In the United States, as 77 million baby boomers approach their sixties and seventies, the number of people over sixty is expected to double from 35 million to 71 million by 2030, and the number of people over age eighty is expected to reach 19.5 million.[1]

As a result, more people than ever before are now or will soon be caring for elderly family members at home. Studies show that 29 percent of the country's adult population—almost 65.7 million people—are caregivers.[2] There's even a term, the "sandwich generation," for people who are looking after kids and parents at the same time. Although there's no doubt it's difficult to grow old, caring for aging family members takes its physical, emotional, and financial tolls on caregivers too.

In this chapter, you'll find touch-therapy remedies with stress-relieving benefits that can soothe not only your elderly loved ones, but caregivers and active seniors as well. They're gentle, noninvasive, safe, and very effective for calming the body and the mind.

Benefits for Caregivers

One of the most important touch-therapy benefits for caregivers is its ability to help you switch from "work mode" to the present moment, so that you can experience an emotional connection with the person you're caring for. Dealing with the pain of others on a daily basis is difficult, and it can be extremely demanding if you have other obligations that require your attention. Touch can help you forget about what's going on around you, all the problems and worries of your day, and help you tune into the person in front of you. Even if it's just for a few minutes, you become 100 percent present with that other person, so you can connect on a deeper level. Through touch, you can show your compassion, understanding, and love, which is especially poignant when caring for someone who may have cared for you or your spouse.

Another benefit for caregivers is that whenever you touch someone, the reward center of *your* brain is affected and dopamine, the feel-good chemical, is released in *your* body as well as in the person you are touching. If you've ever held hands with an older person and seen his or her face light up with happiness, you know how that happiness becomes contagious. You can't help but smile along with the person and feel warm and fuzzy inside. Touch works both ways, so that both you and the person you're touching feel good. Touch therapy is a promising intervention that can reduce elderly and caregiver stress at the same time.

Benefits for the Elderly

By gently manipulating the body and stimulating the mind, touch therapy provides the perfect balance needed to improve seniors' health and general well-being. Like eyesight and hearing, our sense of touch is vulnerable to the effects of age and deteriorates as we get older. Starting around the age of eighteen, we lose about 1 percent of our tactile sense every year. "By the time you're old, you've lost a whole lot of the touch sense," says neuroscientist David Linden.[3]

Apparently, the nerve endings in our hands decrease and the nerves die off forever. Also, the myelin coating our nerve fibers, which enables them to communicate quickly with the brain, breaks down, so the information gets to the brain more slowly.[4] This is one reason the elderly are more prone to dropping things and falling. Since elderly people get less tactile information from their sense of touch (particularly on their hands and feet), touch therapy is particularly beneficial because it enhances their awareness of tactile sensations—such as stroking, pressure, movement, and warmth.

Touch therapy for the elderly also promotes relaxation and better sleep, strengthening of muscles while reducing tension, and an increased range of motion; in fact, it helps manage many age-related conditions. Massage boosts circulation, eases stress, and relieves aches and pains, which is important physiologically for people who don't move around much. Studies show that massage can help reduce chronic pain, particularly in joints, such as the shoulder or knee, while also improving stability and posture.[5] This may help decrease falls in older adults. Other studies show massage can help high blood pressure and osteoarthritis.[6]

Researchers believe touch can strengthen the immune system by reducing the stress hormone cortisol. Since elderly people, who could use the immunity-boosting benefits of touch the most, are getting touched the least, it's quite valuable for caregivers to use it more. Studies have shown that even a brief massage can reduce stress levels and agitation behavior in older adults living with dementia, such as physical expressions like pacing and wandering. Massage therapy has also been shown to reduce aggression in Alzheimer's patients and improve those clients' quality of life.[7] Research shows that massage therapy provides clinical benefits to hospice patients, such as decreased pain.[8]

Finally, attentive, nurturing touch establishes an intimate bond that conveys compassion. Many elderly people are isolated, whether it's because they're home alone most of the time or at a nursing home without family nearby to visit, and they're truly touch deprived. Some elderly people have no one at all to care for them, and they crave social connection. Touch literally connects the elderly person to someone else. If you've ever visited a nursing home, you've probably witnessed the depressing reality of patients left alone sitting in wheelchairs or in their beds for hours on end. Even if they're living at home with family, older people can still feel lonely, because they're missing the independence and interaction they had when they were able to drive or work outside of the home. Touch can help alleviate feelings of loneliness, which if ignored, can lead to depression, irritability, and lack of interest in life.[9]

By incorporating touch therapy into a regular health-care routine for the elderly, their quality of life is greatly increased, which helps them to feel healthier and happier. Touch therapy is an easy and affordable way for caregivers to promote better health for the millions of older people being cared for at home as well as the 1.5 million patients in over sixteen thousand elder-care residences.

Benefits for Active Seniors

Touch therapy offers active seniors who care for themselves a way to be proactive in nurturing their own physical and emotional health and improving and prolonging their quality of life. They can reap the benefits of touch before reaching a stage of life when they may require more help or lose their independence. Active seniors who live with partners or family can take advantage of the mutual benefits that touch brings by massaging each other. For example, a study at Miami's Touch Research Institute reported that elderly individuals who volunteered to give massages to infants had less anxiety and depression, lower stress hormones, and enhanced well-being.[10]

According to Nancy M. Porambo, president of the American Massage Therapy Association (AMTA), "The aging of both the silent and boomer generations calls for an increased focus on improving and prolonging quality of life in this population. While integrating massage therapy into a health and wellness plan is useful for all ages, it holds particular value in the growing elder population."[11] With our unprecedented longevity (seventy-eight years is the average life span in the United States), we should do everything in our power to assure that our quality of life complements our length of life. As Erdman Palmore, a professor emeritus at Duke University who has written more than a dozen books on aging, says, "One can say unequivocally that older people are getting smarter, richer, and healthier as time goes on."[12]

The New and Improved Over-Fifty Mind-set

Today older people are taking better care of themselves than ever before, and one of the ways they're doing this is through *touch*. According to the National Center for Health Statistics, approximately nine million people over the age of fifty-five received a total of thirty-nine million massages in twelve months (54 percent for medical reasons and 23 percent for stress).[13] As baby boomers age, many of those who already use massage will continue to do so, while others may seek it out for the first time as a way to relieve stress and achieve the best health possible. Being proactive about health in older age is vital, since we live in a culture that worships youth and views aging as a stigma, and that affects health care. In fact, the elderly are less likely to receive preventive care and often lack access to doctors trained in their needs.[14] Touch therapy is a particularly effective stress-prevention and stress-management tool for seniors.

The Techniques

Touch-therapy techniques for the elderly are modified massage techniques that take into account age-related conditions, such as pain, lack of mobility, and thin skin more prone to tearing and bruising. The techniques for seniors are much more gentle, use less pressure, and usually incorporate stretching. They're all safe for older individuals.

TIPS FOR WORKING WITH THE ELDERLY

- *Pay attention to reactions:* As always, communicate as much as possible and watch how the person you're touching is reacting. This is extremely important when touching the elderly.
- *Use light pressure:* Keep your pressure light, particularly when you are stroking away from the heart. Ideally, you want to encourage the circulation to move in the direction of the heart by applying firmer pressure as you stroke toward the heart.
- *Do shorter sessions:* Five minutes may be enough for the elderly. Be conscious of how the person you are touching is feeling (ask!) and adjust your timing accordingly.

COLD SENSITIVITY SWEDISH MASSAGE REMEDY

"I'm always cold!" is a common complaint of many older people who suffer from increased sensitivity to the cold, particularly in their hands and feet. They may complain that they're cold all the time, even when the temperature is mild. This could be a sign of a medical problem like diabetes (which actually decrease sensitivity in the extremities) or hypertension, but there are many other possible reasons, including drugs, for a reduction in blood circulation and an increase in heat loss. High cholesterol as well as thyroid conditions can also reduce blood flow and affect people's ability to regulate their temperature. In fact, as people age, their metabolic responses to the cold may be slower. Studies have shown that older people are more likely to have slightly colder body temperatures than younger people.[15]

This Cold Sensitivity Massage Remedy uses Swedish massage strokes to increase circulation to the arms and legs, which warms up the body quickly. The strokes are long and smooth, with pressure moving toward the heart. I like

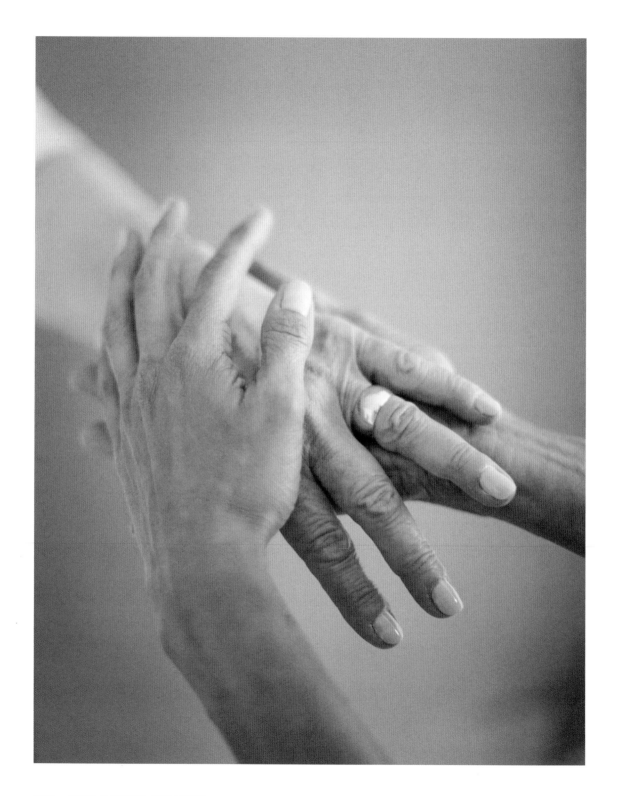

to use natural oil with a few drops of clove oil in it to really warm the skin. However, if the person is sensitive to fragrance, be safe and stick to unscented oil or a scent that you know he or she likes.

1. Warm some oil or lotion in your hands, and start with either the legs or the arms. The strokes are the same for both limbs. If you begin with the arms, do both arms, then switch to legs, and do both legs. (Do *not* do arm, leg, arm, leg—it can feel very unsettling!)

2. *Effleurage:* Assuming you start with the arms, take one arm in your hands (you may have to adjust clothing) and slowly stroke with both hands from the fingertips all the way up to the shoulder, around the top of the arm, and all the way back down, stroking your hands along the underside of the arm. Use light pressure, and use the first few strokes to spread the oil or lotion. Repeat this effleurage stroke several times, increasing your pressure as you stroke up the arm and decreasing pressure as you stroke back down to the hand.

3. *Petrissage:* Next, apply pressure with your thumb on the top of the forearm and the rest of your fingers underneath and stroke from the wrist to the elbow with one hand, and with the other hand stroke from the elbow to the wrist; your hands will be on either side of the person's forearm. Continue this stroke several times, alternating hands. This is called petrissage, and it greatly improves circulation.

4. *Effleurage:* Return to the first effleurage stroke, moving from the hand to the shoulder and back down. Do this several times.

5. *Feathering:* Finish by using your fingertips to lightly stroke down from the shoulder to the fingers, hand over hand, several times. This is called feathering.

6. Repeat on the other arm.

7. Switch to the legs and repeat all of the above strokes on the legs. The order is: effleurage, petrissage (from ankle to knee, then knee to hip), effleurage, feathering.

COLD FEET (POOR CIRCULATION)
REFLEXOLOGY REMEDY

Poor circulation in the feet and legs, also known as peripheral vascular disease (PVD), is a very common problem for the aged population. It occurs when the arteries supplying blood to the limbs are damaged, as in atherosclerosis.

Lack of physical activity, diabetes, high blood pressure, high cholesterol, and other neuropathies are also associated with poor circulation to the feet. When this happens, people often complain of tingling, coldness, lack of feeling in their feet, and, as a result, a lack of balance when they walk. They may also have swelling from edema, cramps, and pain. Reflexology is a great way to wake up the feet and improve blood circulation and lymph flow to the rest of the body, which is particularly helpful for people with poor mobility. It's one of the easiest and most acceptable ways to begin touching someone who is not used to being touched.

1. Make sure the person is comfortable, with feet propped up so you can easily reach them.

2. Before beginning, I recommend taking two warm, wet washcloths and wrapping them around the person's feet for a few minutes. This serves two purposes: it cleans the feet, and it warms them so that energy begins to flow.

3. Begin by warming your hands by rubbing them together. Then take one foot in your hands. (It helps if you're comfortably seated either in a chair in front of or on the bed next to the person.) Gently bend the foot forward and flex it back a few times; then rotate the foot clockwise a few times and then reverse.

4. Using lotion or oil (or nothing if you prefer), alternately rub your thumbs on the sole of the foot, starting at the heel and moving up toward the toes. Try to cover the entire foot. This stimulates all of the reflex areas.

5. Next, use your thumb to make small circles all over the foot. To stimulate specific reflex areas that correspond to parts of the body where the person has existing problems, look at the reflexology chart on p. 21. Spend several minutes applying static pressure and then making small circles in both directions on selected areas to release congested energy.

6. Place your palms on the sides of each foot and gently roll the foot between your hands.

7. Take each toe between your thumb and index finger and rub from the base of the toe to the toenail. Then gently pull outward so you sort of snap the toenail between your fingers.

8. Finish by lightly tapping all over the sole of the foot to wake up the nerve endings.

9. Repeat on the other foot.

AROMATHERAPY FOR COLD HANDS AND FEET

3 drops clove oil
3 drops black pepper oil
3 drops ginger oil
2 ounces unscented natural oil

Blend the above oils and place a few drops on the palm of one hand. Rub the oil between your hands for a few seconds until you feel the warmth of these oils between your fingers. As you do the remedies this warmth will penetrate the skin and improve cold hands and feet.

NOTE: *Make sure to wipe the feet after using oil on them or put socks on, so that no one slips!*

THERAPEUTIC-TOUCH REMEDY FOR SENIORS

I recommend this remedy for people who are fragile and need the least invasive therapy. Therapeutic touch is a kind of gentle healing that uses a practice called the "laying on of hands" to balance energy fields. Depending on how frail the elderly person is, you can either lay your hands on the body or just let your hands hover over the body without physically touching it. Therapeutic touch is based on the theory that the body, mind, and emotions form a complex energy field. Good health is an indication of a balanced energy field, while illness represents imbalance. By placing your hands on or near someone's body with the intention to heal, you can help open energy channels, alleviate stress, and enhance a general sense of well-being. You're actually helping the body's own healing mechanisms function.

Studies suggest that therapeutic touch may help to heal wounds, reduce pain, and lessen anxiety.[16] Together with medical treatment, therapeutic touch can help with many additional conditions, including fibromyalgia, sleep apnea, restless-leg syndrome, allergies, bronchitis, lupus, Alzheimer's disease, and other forms of dementia.[17]

There are eight general regions of the body where energy is sensed—the head, throat, heart, stomach, lower abdomen, sacral region, knees, and feet. As you place your hands on or near these areas, you may sense warmth, coolness, static, or tingling over any areas of energy "congestion" or "blockage."

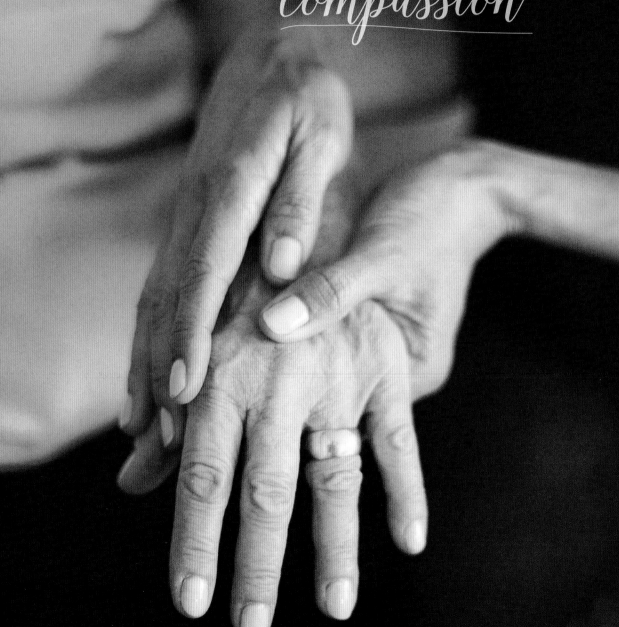

touch is

compassion

All you need to do is keep your hands there for a minute or two, allowing the heat and energy of your hands to transmit to the person you're touching.

Before you begin, I suggest you wash your hands, take a few deep breaths, and clear your mind of anything that may be worrying you. Relax, tune in to the person you're about to touch, and try to remain open to any emotions that come up. Really, there's no right or wrong way to do this. Touch with your hands and your heart, and you're doing it perfectly.

1. Make sure the elderly person is comfortable (sitting or lying down is fine) and warm. You can cover the person with a blanket and lay your hands over the blanket. Suggest that the person take this time to relax, and minimize any talking, so he or she can tune in to feeling.

2. Begin by rubbing your hands together to create warmth and energy.

3. Since feet are the least vulnerable parts of the body, I usually begin at the feet and work up the body, finishing at the head. However, use your own intuition and place your hands wherever you feel they should go. Place your hands on an area and hold them there for 2 to 3 minutes, which may seem like a long time, but it's *very* relaxing. People usually zone out after a few minutes. As you move to the next area, shake the energy off your hands and then rub them together again to create more warmth.

4. These are the areas you should try to cover: feet, knees, lower back (you can slip your hands under the back if the person is lying flat), lower abdomen, stomach, chest, throat, neck, and head.

5. To finish, I like to place one hand on the forehead and one hand on the heart. This connects the heart and mind and is a very soothing position to end with.

6. *Always* wash your hands after therapeutic touch, so you don't take on any of the other person's energy.

LOVE AND COMPASSION ARE NECESSITIES,
NOT LUXURIES. WITHOUT THEM HUMANITY
CANNOT SURVIVE.

—DALAI LAMA

CHAPTER NINE

Healing Remedies

Touch During Illness

When you're sick, there's really nothing more comforting than compassionate touch from someone who cares. Whether it's something as simple as a hand in yours or a gentle shoulder or foot rub, when someone touches you with love and kindness, it can be as healing as chicken soup for your body and soul. This is when you need touch the most.

Yet oftentimes when someone is ill, people around them, including friends and family, don't know what to do to help that person feel better. They may even be afraid to touch sick individuals for fear of hurting them or catching whatever they have, even if it's not contagious. When someone you care about is in any kind of physical or emotional pain, one of the most valuable things to know is that touch has the power to bring relief and consolation. In fact, touch therapy is a vital component of caring for the sick.

As a massage therapist, I've worked with many sick people at home and in hospitals and hospices and witnessed firsthand the power of touch therapy.

In this chapter I'd like to share with you my most effective, gentle, safe, and easy-to-do touch-therapy remedies for relieving discomfort and pain, so that you can offer support to someone you care about. Although I can't cover every illness that exists in just one chapter, I've included specific touch-therapy remedies for some of the most common diseases, including arthritis, cancer, diabetes, digestive disorders (stomach pain, constipation, reflux, irritable bowel syndrome, Crohn's disease, and ulcerative colitis), and fibromyalgia. The remedies for each illness are different, but the techniques are all extremely gentle and can, in fact, be used interchangeably on anyone who is sick. However, if you want the most appropriate remedy for an illness, I suggest following the instructions under that specific illness.

Recently there has been a lot of new research on massage therapy for people with illnesses, and massage is increasingly recognized as an alternative medical treatment. According to a recent consumer survey sponsored by the American Massage Therapy Association, 77 percent of respondents said their primary reason for receiving a massage in the past year was medical or stress-related.[1] When used in combination with standard care, massage can help reduce stress, anxiety, pain, and fatigue and can help increase quality of life.[2]

Studies suggest that massage therapy can improve the emotional and physical well-being of patients with serious illnesses, including cancer, and late-stage diseases. New research shows that massage is helpful for manually controlling symptoms in people suffering from metastatic cancer and rheumatoid arthritis as well as post-cardiac surgery pain and Lyme disease.[3] Another study suggests that massage therapy is able to increase quality of life and decrease pain for fibromyalgia sufferers.[4]

By using simple touch-therapy techniques you can actually change the lives of those with serious illnesses by making the unbearable bearable. For example, difficult treatments such as chemotherapy can be less stressful when touch is involved. Studies show that simply holding someone's hand, even a stranger's, can lower stress levels.[5] It makes sense that after so much poking and prodding during medical treatments, the gentleness of touch can bring much-needed stress relief. It's important to note that when people are sick, they may feel vulnerable and less keen on being touched. I promise that these touch-therapy techniques are the least invasive, yet most soothing. I suggest starting by just placing your hands on someone for a minute or two, and chances are that soon enough they'll welcome a massage from you.

Throughout this book I talk a lot about how stress can cause illness, yet it's important to realize that the reverse is also true: battling any illness causes its own kind of anxiety and stress. In addition to physically painful and distressing symptoms, illness can bring about uncomfortable emotions including anger, sadness, frustration, and depression, which can cause people to isolate themselves and disengage from the people close to them. Touch therapy can help you connect with those who may be in the midst of emotional turmoil and have pulled away emotionally or physically. The remedies in this chapter can help you nurture them, so they feel they're not alone on their journey to better health. And by nurturing someone else, you'll find that you feel rewarded as well, for you cannot touch someone without being touched yourself.

I'll never forget the emotions that surfaced in me several years ago when my dad got sick suddenly and almost died. He was in the hospital for many weeks. Every few hours I would massage his feet and hands, which were numb due to an undiagnosed neuropathy and spinal stenosis. Besides distracting my dad from the relentless pain that he was in, these moments of physical closeness and energetic exchange were some of the most intimate and memorable of my life. Even with nurses and doctors buzzing in and out of the room, I could sense that my dad felt cared for and loved when I touched him. Massage empowered me with a physical way to help my dad at a time when I thought there was nothing else I could do.

Over the years I've taught many workshops on healing techniques for caregivers and family members of people with cancer as well as self-massage techniques for people going through cancer treatment. At City of Hope, a leading comprehensive cancer center in Los Angeles, I led a workshop on reflexology techniques to relieve the symptoms of cancer treatment. The room was filled with patients, nurses, spouses of patients undergoing chemotherapy, a mother whose son was undergoing radiation, and even a nun. At the end of the class, I asked everyone to write down the most valuable thing they learned. What surprised me the most was that, rather than indicate a specific technique, almost everyone stated in one way or another that the most valuable thing was the feeling of being empowered and inspired to touch more. The most moving response came from the mother, who said, "Thank you. I'm less afraid to touch my son now."

Considering the impersonal nature of today's health-care system, my experience working with people who are sick has made it clear to me that the importance of simple touch cannot be overlooked. Whether you use these touch remedies at home or in a health-care environment, by combining your compassionate presence with touch-therapy techniques you'll be able to effectively soothe and support someone you care about who's dealing with an illness. The most important thing to remember is to listen with sensitivity, using your eyes, ears, hands, and heart. Try to give every person you touch your undivided attention and compassion. Even if you find yourself simply sitting next to someone and holding hands, just remember that healing the body is linked with healing the soul. Touching with your hands and your heart can be a powerful healing tool for helping those you love.

GUIDELINES FOR WORKING WITH THOSE WHO ARE ILL

- Always ask if the person would like a massage before beginning.
- Make sure the person you are about to touch is comfortable and warm.
- Remember, this is gentle massage, never deep massage.
- Consult a physician to determine the advisability of massage.

When Not to Use Touch Therapy

Touch therapy is noninvasive, gentle, and safe to use. However, it is not recommended when the following are present:

- Fever
- Contagious diseases, including any cold or flu
- Skin diseases

Medical Contraindications

For some conditions it is advisable to consult a physician for approval before using touch therapy. These conditions do not necessarily mean that touch therapy is a no-go. In fact, massage is very therapeutic for many medical conditions. It's just best to get approval from a physician. These include:

- Cardio-vascular conditions (thrombosis, phlebitis, hypertension, heart conditions)
- Edema
- Psoriasis or eczema
- High blood pressure
- Osteoporosis
- Cancer
- Nervous or psychotic conditions
- Heart problems, angina, pacemakers
- Neuritis
- Epilepsy
- Diabetes
- Bell's palsy, trapped or pinched nerves

Arthritis

Today in the United States an estimated 52.5 million adults suffer from arthritis and approximately 294,000 children under age eighteen (1 in 250 children) have been diagnosed with arthritis or another rheumatologic condition. Arthritis is inflammation of one or more of your joints, and the main symptoms are joint pain, stiffness, swelling, redness, and decreased range of motion, which typically worsen with age. Arthritis includes more than 100 different rheumatic diseases and conditions, the most common of which is osteoarthritis, a degenerative joint disease that affects about 33 million Americans.[6] Studies show that massage with moderate pressure can improve symptoms of rheumatoid arthritis, resulting specifically in less pain, greater grip strength, and improved range of motion in the upper limbs.[7] Another study shows that neck arthritis pain is reduced and range of motion is increased by massage therapy.[8] The techniques are simple and some (the arm and shoulder technique) can be done to yourself, as the participants in the rheumatoid arthritis study were taught self-massage.

ARTHRITIC ARMS AND SHOULDERS MASSAGE REMEDY

1. *Effleurage:* Warm a small amount of oil or lotion in your hands and stroke from the top of the wrist to the shoulder with moderate pressure, then from the shoulder back to the wrist. On the top of the hand, stroke from the wrist to the tips of the fingers and back to the wrist. Repeat on the underside of the arm. Do this several times for each arm.

2. *Milking:* Starting at the top of the arm, gently squeeze the arm between your fingers and thumb as you gradually move down to the wrist and back up to the shoulder from the wrist. Continue to apply moderate pressure. Switch hands so that you're holding the arm with your other hand, and repeat on the other side.

3. *Friction:* Make circular movements with four fingers on top of the arm, moving across the shoulder and down the arm and top of hand. Repeat on underside of arm.

NOTE: *You can also use these strokes on the legs to relieve arthritic pain.*

ARTHRITIC HAND
MASSAGE REMEDY
....

I. No oil or lotion is needed. Using
your index finger and thumb, apply
pressure to the base of one finger on
both sides and make small circles.
Continue this as you move up the
finger to the tip, and then all the way
down to the wrist. (I like to begin
with the thumb and progress to the
pinkie.)

2. Repeat on every finger.

3. Next, hold the thumbnail between
your index finger and thumb (thumb
on top). Rub the finger in the di-
rection of the wrist, making small rubs as you move toward the wrist.
Repeat on every finger.

4. Finish by interlocking your fingers and gently bending the wrist forward
and back, and then rotate the wrist in one direction a few times and reverse.

5. Repeat on the other hand.

ARTHRITIC NECK MASSAGE REMEDY
....

I. Position yourself behind the person, who is lying flat on the back (on a
bed or in a recliner is best). Warm some oil or lotion in your hands and
place your hands under the neck, at the base of the skull, with your fingertips resting on the muscles on either side of the spine.

2. Apply moderate pressure with your fingertips and slowly pull your hands
toward you, allowing them to follow the contours of the neck. This gives
a nice stretch to the neck and increases circulation. You can alternate
between doing this stroke with both hands together and doing one hand
after the other.

3. Next, reach one hand diagonally underneath the neck and then apply
moderate pressure to the neck as you pull your hand back under the neck.
This will gently turn the head to one side.

4. As one hand is pulling and the head starts to turn, reach your other hand underneath and do the same thing you just did. Continue to alternate hands, gently lifting up the neck and turning the head from side to side.

5. To finish, bring the head back to center and repeat the first stroke you did with both hands lifting up and pulling back toward you.

Cancer

After years of experience working with cancer patients, I know, and now research offers proof, that gentle touch therapies are safe and extremely beneficial for people with cancer. Along with emotional support and comfort, there are real physical benefits that come from touch before, during, and after treatments. According to the American Cancer Center, studies[9] show that massage can decrease many cancer-related symptoms and the side effects of treatment, such as stress, nausea, fatigue, muscle tension, depression, anxiety, insomnia, and pain.

Massage also helps to boost your "natural killer cells," the immune system's first line of defense against invading illness. Natural killer cells (also called NK cells) are a type of white blood cell that helps boost the immune system. According to Tiffany Fields, "We know that cortisol destroys natural killer cells. Therefore, since massage decreases cortisol, your immune cells get a boost." Massage even seems to boost immunity in people with severely compromised immune systems, such as breast-cancer patients. And perhaps most important, massage has led cancer patients to report an increased sense of well-being.[10]

In a five-year NIH-funded study on the effects of reflexology and cancer, researchers at the University of Michigan found that out of 385 women with advanced-stage breast cancer and on chemotherapy, reflexology improved physical function by 10 percent. The improvements reflected a better ability to walk, carry groceries, and climb stairs.[11]

In a five-week study at the University of Miami, massage therapy and progressive muscle-relaxation therapy were compared in fifty-eight women with stages I and II breast cancer. Both groups reported feeling less anxious, *and* the massage group also reported feeling less depressed. The massage group also showed increased levels of a brain chemical called dopamine, which helps produce a feeling of well-being. In addition, for the massage group, there was an increase in natural killer cells from the first to the last day of the study.[12]

Today, many health-care professionals recognize massage as a useful, noninvasive addition to standard medical treatment, and more hospitals are starting to include massage therapy in their integrative medicine programs as an adjunct therapy to cancer treatment. As Hollye Jacobs, cancer survivor and author of the *New York Times* bestselling book *The Silver Lining: A Supportive and Insightful Guide to Breast Cancer,* says:

> During my treatment for breast cancer, touch therapy was an integral part of my care. Massage and reflexology not only relieved many of my (horrendous!) side effects, but they also provided me with the comfort and strength to get through some of the most difficult of circumstances. I hired my practitioners based on referrals from my cancer center and their experience with other cancer patients. I talked with my health-care team about the safety and timing of each to ensure that these therapies were coordinated into my overall plan of care. Based on my experience, I highly recommend that everyone incorporate touch therapy into the cancer treatment and recovery process.[13]

One of my projects that I'm most excited about is the in-hospital massage program I'm developing at City of Hope, a leading comprehensive cancer center in Los Angeles. My goal is to develop a program that offers touch-therapy services to both in- and out-patients as well as to family members and caregivers of cancer patients. The program will also include workshops that teach simple and safe techniques that patients can do to themselves and soothing techniques that caregivers can do bedside.

Normally, one of the first things people ask me when discussing touch therapy for oncology is: "Is it safe?" And the answer is *yes*! Of course, you should always consult your physician. But rest assured, these touch-therapy techniques, which involve no physical manipulation or deep pressure, are extremely gentle and safe to use on everyone.

GUIDELINES FOR WORKING WITH CANCER PATIENTS

- Do not use deep pressure. Always use light to moderate pressure.
- Never massage at the site of a tumor.
- Avoid massaging areas that are sensitive due to radiation.
- Avoid massage if the person has lymphedema (instead, use the Therapeutic-Touch Remedy).
- Ask about any sensitive body areas, if there are areas that, if touched, would feel uncomfortable, and if the pressure you are using feels okay.
- Occasionally, chemotherapy will cause extra sensitivity in the feet, so before you begin, always ask about any tender areas and avoid those areas.

- Ask the person about preferences for your use of lotion, oil, or nothing. Also ask if the person is sensitive to smells, as chemotherapy can cause people to have more sensitivity to odors. I generally stick to unscented lotion (which is less messy than oil) and add a few drops of a calming essential oil, such as lavender, only if the person wants it.
- Make sure you wash your hands before touching anyone.

FOOT REFLEXOLOGY REMEDY FOR CANCER PATIENTS

I typically start with the feet, because they're usually the least vulnerable part of the body, and a foot massage can really help someone who's going through treatment feel grounded and safe. If possible, I like to have people soak their feet in warm water with 2 cups of Epsom salts for 10 to 15 minutes. This really helps them loosen up and "tune out" before a treatment.

1. Make sure the person is comfortable, with the feet propped up on a bed or chair so you can easily reach them.

2. Warm your hands by rubbing them together and then take one foot in your hands. Slowly bend the foot forward and flex it back; then rotate it in one direction and then the other. Bend the toes backward and forward a few times.

3. Rub some lotion or oil between your palms (or use nothing, if you prefer) and gently stroke over the entire foot, top and bottom, to warm it up. Use the palms of your hands to apply light pressure to the soles of the feet; then make circles in one direction for 10 to 15 seconds, and then in the other.

4. Bring your thumbs to the heel of the foot and alternate rubbing one thumb and then the other in an upward motion.

5. Next, thumb-walk over the entire sole of the foot, starting at the heel and moving up to the base of the toes. This stimulates all of the reflexology points.

6. Using your thumb, make small circles along the inner edge of the foot, close to the middle of the foot, and covering about 1½ inches in toward the center of the foot. Spend a minute or two here. This is the reflex area to the stomach and stimulating this part of the foot can help relieve and prevent nausea.

7. Move your thumbs to the outer edge of the foot, just below the pinkie toe,

and make circles in this area from the base of the pinkie to about 2 inches below it. This is the reflex area to the shoulders and stimulating here can release tension and help fatigue.

8. Pinch each toe between your thumb and index finger to stimulate the sinuses and finish at the big toe. Hold the fleshy part of the big toe (behind the nail) for 10 to 15 seconds with firm pressure, and then make small circles in one direction, then the other, maintaining firm pressure between your thumb and finger. This is the reflex area to the brain and this can relieve and prevent headaches as well as calm anxiety.

9. Repeat on the other foot.

HAND REFLEXOLOGY REMEDY FOR CANCER PATIENTS

1. Sit comfortably next to the person and take one hand between your hands. I usually spend 10 to 20 seconds just holding the hand, in silence, without moving, because it helps me become fully present with that person and it helps them relax. As the person's hand warms up in yours, you'll feel any tension or rigidity in the hand decrease.

2. Warm a small amount of lotion in your hands and then gently spread the lotion over the person's entire hand by alternating your hands. Carefully pull each finger. Then interlace your hand with the other person's, so that the palm of the person's hand is facing up and the fingers are spread out.

3. With fingers interlaced, use your thumbs to walk over the entire palm, starting at the wrist and moving up to the base of the fingers. This stimulates all of the reflexology points.

4. Focus on the center of the hand, which is the reflex area to the solar plexus, and make small circles in one direction for 10 seconds, then in the other. This can relieve anxiety and calm the body and mind.

5. Follow the reflexology chart (p. 21) and make small circles on the reflex areas for the stomach (to help nausea) and the spine (to help backaches from sitting or lying in one position).

6. Finally, pinch the tip of the thumb between your index finger and thumb to stimulate the reflex area to the brain. This can relieve headaches.

7. Repeat on the other hand.

THERAPEUTIC-TOUCH REMEDY FOR CANCER PATIENTS

There may be times when patients are so ill that they don't want any pressure on their body. However, they still want and need touch more than ever. Therapeutic touch is the perfect therapy for someone in this condition, because it's a noninvasive energy therapy that requires little to no contact, yet it promotes healing and reduces pain and anxiety. It's a 100 percent safe, valuable therapy to use if you have any apprehension about touching someone who is ill.

Many years ago I worked with a client during the final months of her struggle with brain cancer. She was very frail, so we decided that I would use therapeutic touch to help her relax. As she lay on the massage table, I would alternate laying my hands very lightly on different parts of her body and then allowing them to hover about an inch above the skin. I always started at her feet and slowly progressed up to her head, where I let my hands hover around her ears, face, and skull. I remember she used to tell me that after a few minutes all she felt was warmth moving up her body and by the end she was totally relaxed. She told me that these treatments were the only times she could easily fall into a deep sleep. Even though it seemed as if not much was happening on the outside, I could tell by her reaction at the end of each session that something significant was happening on the inside. This, my friends, is the beauty of therapeutic touch.

1. Rub your hands together to create heat and then shake them out to get rid of any negative energy.

2. Make sure the person is lying flat and is covered by a blanket to stay warm. You can lay your hands on the blanket or reach underneath to lay your hands directly on the skin.

3. Stand at the person's feet and place the palms of your hands on the tops of the feet. Hold them here for 1 minute, then lift them 1 inch above and hold for another minute.

4. Repeat on the soles of the feet, then on various parts of the body as you slowly progress toward the head; touch the legs, stomach, shoulders, arms, and chest. Use your intuition and stay longer on areas to which you feel drawn. There's no right or wrong way to do this. Simply think of yourself as an open channel of energy, getting rid of anything negative and allowing only positive energy to flow.

5. When you reach the head, spend a minute or two with your hands on and above the neck, the skull, the ears, the eyes, and the cheeks.

6. To finish, use your fingertips to lightly brush 1 inch above the skin from the head down to the neck. I think of this as brushing any negative energy out of the person through the feet.

7. If the person has fallen asleep, do not wake!

Diabetes

Touch therapy can have a profound effect on people with diabetes, a metabolic disease that affects over sixteen million people in the United States. Whether it's type 1 or type 2 diabetes, living with this disease is inherently stressful. The body's inability to produce any or enough insulin causes elevated levels of glucose in the blood. The tremendous strain on the body's systems combined with emotional anxiety can lead to fatigue, poor circulation, and many other complications, including damage to the eyes, kidneys, heart, blood vessels, and nervous system.[14] In addition, the elevated blood sugars can lead to a thickening of the fascia surrounding the muscles and organs, which often results in pain and stiffness around the joints.

Massage has been recommended for diabetes for nearly a hundred years.[15] Studies show that massage decreases anxiety in diabetics and calms their nervous system.[16] It decreases the production of stress hormones, which is beneficial to blood sugar levels.[17] It also increases the circulation of blood and lymph, which improves the transport of oxygen and other nutrients into the body's tissues, and encourages more efficient uptake of insulin by the cells. Since circulation is often impaired in diabetics, massage is quite beneficial. It can counter the effects of stiffness in muscles, tendons, and ligaments as well as decreased range of motion in the joints.

NOTE: *Changes in blood glucose levels can and do occur when people with diabetes receive massage. Always communicate with the person you are touching and notice any changes in their manner or appearance.*

TRIGGER-POINT REMEDY FOR DIABETICS

Trigger-point therapy, also called myofascial release, is very helpful for diabetics who have pain and stiffness caused by muscle tissue that is tough, fibrous, and inelastic due to thickening of the fascia surrounding the muscles and organs (a direct result of elevated blood sugars). Myofascial trigger points are hypersensitive areas of the body that cause pain in other parts of the body when they are stimulated. By pressing on specific trigger points, you can release tension and

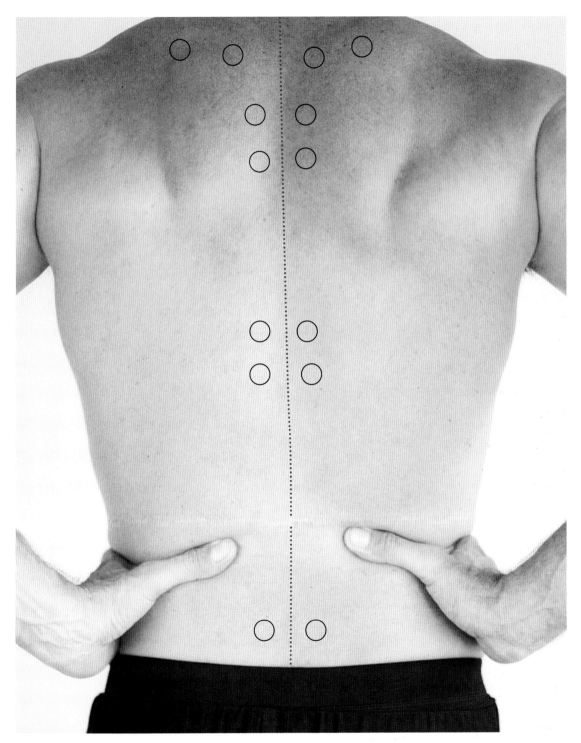

Trigger Points for Diabetes

increase circulation to areas of the body that may be numb or stiff. There's an association between diabetes and trigger points, particularly the trigger point called "diabetic capsulitis," which is associated with the condition "frozen shoulder," frequently diagnosed in diabetics. Follow this simple guide to stimulating the body's potent trigger points and you can increase circulation and relieve pain and stiffness.

I. Have the person lie facedown on the floor, or on a bed with the head close to the end of the bed, so that you can reach the back. Turn the head to one side, so the person is comfortable. This can be done with clothes on.

2. Following the trigger-point chart shown on p. 209, apply firm, static pressure with your thumbs to each point along both sides of the spine for 10 seconds. Begin with the points at the top of the shoulders and work your way down to the points just above the hips. As you apply pressure, ask the person if the pressure is okay and if he or she is feeling any tenderness or pain. If so, lighten your pressure slightly. Repeat two times.

3. Have the person turn over onto the back and use your thumbs to apply firm, static pressure to the points on the front of the body (directly opposite the points you pressed on the back). Press just below the collarbone, in the middle of the chest, a few inches above the belly button and a few inches below the belly button for 10 seconds each. Repeat two times.

Digestive Problems

Digestive problems, such as stomach pain, constipation, reflux, heartburn, irritable bowel syndrome, Crohn's disease, and ulcerative colitis, are all too common in our stressed-out society. Approximately 70 million Americans have digestive disorders, which prompt nearly 60 million visits to doctors' offices and hospitals each year.[18] Although they can affect people of any age, many of these problems occur more frequently as we get older. Unfortunately, these digestive difficulties can be awkward to discuss in polite company, so many people are left to suffer in silence. Touch therapy offers many solutions that you can do to yourself or to someone else to relieve and prevent discomfort and pain.

Research has shown that therapeutic-massage techniques may be helpful for digestive disorders.[19] For example, abdominal massage is helpful immediately after a colonoscopy procedure to eliminate the air that was used to inflate the colon (also called the large intestine) during the examination. Massage has also been shown to help patients after colectomy surgery, in which all or part of the colon is removed. Further research indicates that massage can decrease postoperative pain of all types, decrease doses of analgesics, and increase levels of calmness and feelings of well-being.[20]

Here's a simple remedy you can do to stimulate the spontaneous movement of the digestive tract (a process called peristalsis) and reduce symptoms such as cramping, bloating, gas, and constipation.

NOTE: *Do not use massage during an active flare-up of ulcerative colitis or Crohn's disease, as it can exacerbate the pain. It should be used during periods of remission when pain is not present.*

DIGESTIVE MASSAGE REMEDY

1. Have the person lie on the back on a flat surface (floor or bed) with shirt rolled up, so you can access the stomach. Sit or kneel to one side of the person, and warm some oil or lotion in your hands.

2. Place one hand just below the rib cage (perpendicular to the body) and your other hand just below the belly button. Apply very light pressure and slowly begin to circle your hands in a clockwise direction (never counterclockwise) around the belly button. Try to maintain continuous contact and massage a full circle by lifting hand over hand. Do this for 1 to 2 minutes.

3. Next, with your hands still perpendicular to the person's body and fingers pointing toward each other, begin to stroke down from the bottom of the rib cage to the bottom of the belly. Apply a little more pressure as you "scoop" down the belly, and then lighten your pressure as you scoop up toward the pelvis. Repeat for 20 to 30 seconds.

4. Place your index and middle fingers at the base of the right side of the person's rib cage. Massage small circles moving across the bottom of the rib cage toward the person's left side, then straight down to the bottom of the belly. At the bottom of the belly, massage a squiggly line from the person's left side across to the right, ending at the bottom of the belly on the right side.

5. Starting here, continue to make small circles with your index and middle fingers. Move straight up from the person's lower right side to the bottom of the rib cage, across the rib cage to the left side, down to the lower left belly, and then a squiggly line back across to the right side. Repeat two or three times.

6. Rest your hands to the left and right of the belly button, and just hold them there for at least 20 seconds, allowing the warmth of your hands to penetrate into the belly. Tell the person to take a few deep breaths. Move your hands so they cover the other sides of the belly button. Request a few more deep breaths. This is very soothing to the digestive system.

Fibromyalgia

More than six million Americans (over 90 percent are women) suffer from fibromyalgia, a chronic syndrome characterized by widespread pain, numbness, joint stiffness, intense fatigue, sleep alterations, headaches, spastic colon, anxiety, depression, and sensitivity to bright lights, loud noises, and strong odors. Although the causes are unknown, many people associate the development of fibromyalgia with a physically or emotionally stressful or traumatic event, such as an automobile accident. Some connect it to repetitive injuries or an illness, while for others it seems to occur spontaneously.[21] If you're one of the many suffering from fibromyalgia, new research shows that massage therapy can help. A 2011 study suggests that massage therapy is able to lower anxiety levels, improve quality of sleep, decrease pain, and increase quality of life for fibromyalgia sufferers.[22] The study found reductions in sensitivity to pain at tender points in patients with fibromyalgia.

Since many fibromyalgia sufferers complain of sharper levels of pain in the neck and back, this Swedish massage remedy focuses on these areas of the body.

FIBROMYALGIA MASSAGE REMEDY

I. Have the person lie facedown on a bed, with the head at the foot of the bed, so that you can stand facing the back. You can do this with clothes on or with a bare back, in which case you should use oil or lotion, so you don't pull on the skin.

2. Place your palms on the lower back, on either side of the spine (*not* on the spine), so that your fingers point out toward the side. Lean forward so that the weight of your body puts pressure on the muscles on the sides of the spine, then lift your hands up, move them up the spine about 2 inches, and repeat applying pressure. Continue this all the way up to the base of the neck.

3. Next, place the fingers of both hands on the lower back, on either side of the spine. Apply moderate pressure and gently wiggle your fingers up the back all the way to the base of the skull.

4. Place both hands on the lower back and massage circles on the entire area of the back. Bring your fingertips to either side of the neck, close to the spine, and massage circles from the base of the neck to the base of the skull.

5. Move around to the side of the body and place the palms of both hands on the lower back, perpendicular to the spine. Move one hand forward and the other hand back so that your hands massage in opposite directions across the spine.

6. Finish by placing the palms of your hands on the shoulders and pressing forward slightly, so the neck and shoulders get a nice stretch.

The act of massage unites heaven and earth, spirit and matter, divine and mundane.

—GAYLE MACDONALD, AUTHOR OF *Medicine Hands*

AROMATHERAPY FOR ILLNESS

6 drops clary sage oil
3 drops lavender oil
2 drops lemon oil
2 ounces unscented natural oil

Sometimes when people are sick they become extra sensitive to smells and even the most subtle aromatherapy scents can cause nausea, which is often the case with cancer patients. If you know someone has a smell sensitivity, I suggest using only unscented oil. However, some people love to smell soothing scents when they are sick. This aromatherapy blend is so relaxing that it can take your mind off your body and transport you to a place of peace and tranquility. Simply combine the oils, rub a few drops between your hands, and use the remedies as directed.

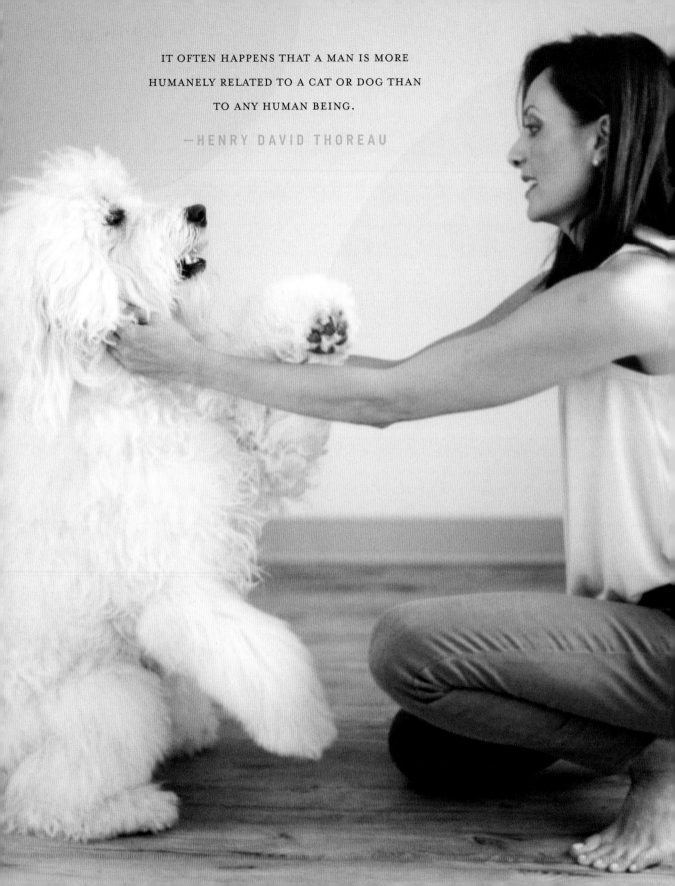

IT OFTEN HAPPENS THAT A MAN IS MORE
HUMANELY RELATED TO A CAT OR DOG THAN
TO ANY HUMAN BEING.

—HENRY DAVID THOREAU

CHAPTER TEN

Kneaded Pets

Pets Need Touch Too

In the stress-filled world we live in, there's no question that our animal friends, who are sensitive by nature, absorb some of the tension and chaos that swirls around them. Pets are like family. They are so in tune to what's going on with us, their owners, that they can sense our emotions just by our tone of voice and body language. They can tell if we're happy or sad, angry or depressed, and everything in between.

There are even special service dogs who are aware of specific conditions, such as when someone is about to have a seizure, and can alert their owners before it happens. In fact, approximately 15 percent of all dogs are naturally able to predict seizures 10 to 20 minutes before they occur, giving the person with the seizure disorder an opportunity to take medication or call for help.[1] Some dogs can even sniff out cancer in the body before it's actually detected! Since 2004, research has begun to accumulate suggesting that dogs may be able to smell the subtle chemical differences between healthy and cancerous tissue, including melanoma and cancers of the lung, breast, bladder, and prostate.[2] It's really amazing. There's a reason why we call dogs our best friends! They're our companions, protectors, and comforters, who trust and love us unconditionally.

As with humans, though occasional stress is not harmful, excessive or chronic stress can be damaging to pets, producing the same negative effects in our pets as it does in us. Stress triggers your pet's internal defense mechanisms, increasing heart rate, releasing the stress hormone cortisol into the bloodstream, and raising energy levels to full throttle with a burst of adrenaline that puts your pet on "high alert." This is evident in a persistently skittish cat or hyperactive dog. However, once their energy reserves are gone, these poor animals weaken, their resistance to illness and disease decreases, and they may get sick. (When my husband and I brought our first baby home from the hospital, his endless, nerve-wracking newborn cries freaked out our cat, Elvis, so much that he died a week later. Sure, he was old, but the stress was more than he could take.)

So what can you do to prevent stressed-out pets? Touch them! But don't just pet them or play with them; instead, massage them in a deliberate and focused way that will encourage their muscles to relax, their emotions to calm down, and their spirits to feel your compassion and love. Massage can increase the bond between you and your pet and nurture an incredible closeness and trust.

Studies show that animals need touch as much as we do. Kittens and puppies, like human infants, can waste away if they're not given affectionate contact, even when their needs for warmth and food are met. It seems that their nervous systems require the stimulation from the gentle licks of their mother's tongue.[3] They miss this when they're removed from their mothers soon after birth. In addition, domesticated animals, who spend the majority of their time indoors, miss out on the physical activities of hunting and free play that would normally keep their body toned and fit. Massage offers pets the tactile stimulation they need to thrive.

Benefits for You

Before I launch into the myriad of benefits that touch therapy can bring to your pet, I need to let you know of the tremendous benefits that are available for you too. Today scientists confirm what pet lovers have always known: pets can make your life happier and healthier. Studies show that when you touch your pet, your brain releases the feel-good hormones oxytocin and prolactin, as well as the neurotransmitter and mood-booster dopamine, in the same stress-reducing way I explained in Chapter 2. In fact, just looking at your pet can induce a "hormone loop" in which these calming chemicals are released in not only your body, but your pet's body as well, according to veterinarian Marty Becker, author of "The Healing Power of Pets."[4] The American Heart Association even says that people who own pets of any kind have better cholesterol levels, a lower risk of hypertension, and a lower rate of heart disease than those who don't have pets.[5]

Today, the research confirming the healing power of pets has led thousands of hospitals, nursing homes, rehabilitation facilities, and even colleges to include pet therapy in their health-care practices. Pet therapy, also known as animal-assisted therapy, is now recognized by the National Institute of Mental Health as a type of psychotherapy for treating depression and other mood disorders. Being around pets appears to feed the soul, promoting a sense of emotional connectedness and overall well-being.

In one study, researchers found that postsurgery patients who used pet therapy requested pain medication 28 percent less often than those who did not have access to pets. Patients who use pet therapy seem to breathe more slowly and feel less tense, which reduces their perception of pain.[6] Today, over four hundred colleges in the United States include pet therapy in their preventative health programs to help college students de-stress. How I wish that was available when I went to college!

Benefits for Pets

Besides the important emotional benefits and social interaction between you and your pet, massage provides animals with the same physical benefits as humans, including relief from stress by loosening tense muscles and joints, improving blood circulation, and overall relaxation after a hard day (even if it was spent at the dog park). Massage is particularly beneficial for geriatric and arthritic pets, who suffer from stiff, painful joints. Specifically, pet massage:

- Relaxes sore, stiff muscles
- Relieves lower-back pain, arthritis, and hip dysplasia pain
- Increases joint flexibility and range of motion
- Encourages the release of endorphins (the body's natural painkillers)
- Increases blood and lymph circulation, which helps healing after an injury
- Releases stress and tension, caused by depression and anxiety
- Enhances the immune system
- Improves digestion

- Increases oxygenation into muscles and tissues, which helps muscle spasms
- Helps injury recovery and reduces the risk of injury in high-energy animals
- Reduces post-surgery adhesions and swelling
- Improves performance level and reduces recovery time
- Helps with palliative pet care
- Enhances your pet's sense of well-being and improves overall health[7]

Just a few minutes a day is all it takes to maintain your pet's health and provide soothing stress relief. Your pet will love the extra attention, and you will benefit too. Research shows that people's stress is reduced and blood pressure drops when they pet dogs, particularly if it's a dog they know and love. Dog petting has also been shown to improve immune function and ease pain, or at least the perception of pain.[8] Researchers at the University of Pennsylvania found that people who have suffered a coronary attack are less likely to have a relapse if they have an animal at home to pet. They believe this is the result of a relaxing, beneficial decrease in heart rate, which occurs while a person is stroking a pet.[9] Now that's a real health benefit!

Today, most show dogs are massaged regularly to keep them relaxed, moving comfortably, and focused before entering the ring. It also promotes a close bond between dog and trainer. Although not as many people have horses as pets, psychologists are recognizing the benefits of using horses in their work (called equine therapy) with autistic children, young people with behavioral problems, and adults with depression and addictions.[10]

Equine massage provides horses with all the physiological benefits of massage, but equine therapy offers a way for people, some of whom may be adverse to talk therapies, to express their emotions. Everyone has a reaction to horses; they may love them or fear them, but they always feel something. As herd animals, horses are attuned to stress and body language. They pick up on the way people are feeling and mirror their emotions by reacting in corresponding ways; they may move away from an angry person, follow someone they trust, and be unsettled when sensing fear. Horses actually have a way of revealing and healing emotions that may be repressed. Even some spas, such as Miraval Resort and Spa in Tucson, Arizona, have begun to offer equine therapy programs to guests.

According to horse trainer Frank Levinson, "It has been clinically documented that just being around horses changes human brainwave patterns. We calm down and become more centered and focused when we are with horses. Horses are naturally empathetic."[11] The origins of pet massage can be traced back to equine massage, which was popularized in the 1970s and 1980s by Jack Meagher, a massage therapist who worked with the U.S. equestrian team. By the early 1990s, a handful of people experienced in human and equine massage began adapting his technique for use on dogs and cats.

Whichever animal you choose to work with, regular massage can strengthen the bond of love and friendship that already exists between you and your pet. When you tune in to the needs and fears of your pet, you begin to understand the subtle body language animals use to communicate with each other and us. There's more to pet massages than just quality time together. It can help with early detection of abnormalities, anything out of the ordinary, such as swelling, fever, weight gain or loss, injury, or painful areas that may signal a health problem. This allows you to seek early treatment before a disease or injury progresses too far. After just a few massages you'll get to know what's normal for your pet's body and you'll have a sense when something changes that may require a trip to the vet. This is one way touch can add to the length and quality of your pet's life.

Massage can also help with physical problems that come with an aging or disabled pet and can improve troublesome behavior such as excitability and nervousness, debilitating fear or shyness, excessive chewing and barking, and aggression. Use massage on a regular basis and you'll be rewarded with a pet that's much more happy, healthy, content, playful, alert, intelligent, responsive, protective, and loving.

What You'll Need

Giving your dog or cat a massage is easy! Unlike massage for humans, pet massage requires no undressing or messy oils. All that's really necessary is a calm, quiet space, a comfortable, firm surface (the floor is great), and your own two hands. Here are some things to keep in mind.

WHEN YOU TOUCH YOUR PET, YOUR BRAIN RELEASES THE FEEL-GOOD HORMONES OXYTOCIN AND PROLACTIN, AS WELL AS THE NEUROTRANSMITTER AND MOOD-BOOSTER DOPAMINE.

- Make sure that both you and your pet are in comfortable positions before starting the massage (the floor is best, or on a table for small animals).
- If you have other animals, try to find a place away from the other animals so your pet is not distracted.
- As puppies and kittens will try to playfully fight with you when you massage them, it's best to massage after they've played and when they are tired.
- Always start with light pressure. The body structure of cats and dogs is much smaller than humans, so even the largest dog requires a lighter touch than people do. Only increase pressure if your pet seems comfortable and reacts positively to deeper strokes.
- Keep in mind that what feels good on you will usually feel good on your pet. For example, animals *love* having their neck, shoulders, and back massaged, because they hold tension there too.
- Maintain a consistent speed, since erratic stroking (fast, then slow, then fast) can cause anxiety and agitate your pet. This is especially important for anxious dogs and cats in general. Aim for one stroke per second so your pet can get used to a rhythm and relax.
- Keep in mind that fast strokes will stimulate and energize, while slow strokes will calm and relax.
- If you hit an area that makes your pet feel vulnerable and tense up, simply lighten your pressure or move to another area of the body.
- Most animals prefer to be massaged on one side of their bodies at a time.
- If you feel any abnormality, such as unusual heat (fever), puffiness, or swelling on the animal, discontinue the massage.
- Never forcibly restrain your pet. If your pet is not into it, try another time.

No Go: When to Avoid Massaging Your Pet

Massage is healing in most circumstances, but you should avoid massage if your pet is suffering from shock, fever, acute inflammation, skin problems, heat stroke, broken bones, ruptured discs, torn muscles, open wounds, surgical sites, or swollen lymph glands (which signal an infection in the body). Also, if your pet seems under the weather, I suggest holding off on massage. Other than that, it's a go!

Getting Started

Whether your goal is therapeutic or you just want to make your pet feel good, massage is a very effective tool for improving health and prolonging life. So go ahead, treat your pet to a soothing rubdown. Spending quality time together may be just what the doctor ordered for you both. Now, if you could just teach your pet to massage *your* neck and shoulders. . . .

RELAXING PET REMEDY

I recommend starting with the Relaxing Pet Remedy because it allows your pet to warm up to your touch. It helps your pet relax and helps you get quiet and centered. This is great for nervous or fearful dogs, and all cats, who need to become accustomed to being handled by humans early on. Gentle massage can help cats who aren't accustomed to touch and improve their socialization. This technique is something you can do anytime your pet is anxious, such as while at the veterinarian or traveling. Your animal will melt in your hands if you keep your pressure steady and slow. Remember, animals pick up our feelings, so you always want to approach your pet as calmly as possible.

1. With your pet lying on one side, place your hands gently but firmly on your pet's head and neck and hold still for a minute or two. This may seem like nothing, but it's actually very calming to the animal, and it helps desensitize ticklish or painful areas before you massage them. During the massage, if you touch an area that seems to be uncomfortable for your pet, just hold your hands still for a moment, and your pet will be more receptive to your touch.

2. Place your palms flat on your pet's head and make long, slow effleurage strokes all the way down the neck, the length of the spine, and the tail. You can stroke both hands together or alternate hands. Keep your hands on the muscles on the sides of the spine, never directly on the spine. Repeat several times, gradually increasing pressure if your pet likes it. With your pet in a side-lying position, first massage the side that is accessible to you and then turn your pet over to do the other side. Focus on what you are feeling and pay attention to all the layers, from hair through skin, fat, muscle, and bone. After a few minutes place one hand at the base of the pet's head and the other on the pelvis, which is the high point over your pet's hips. These two areas correspond to the part of the spinal cord that encourages the "relaxation response."

3. Next, use the same long, gliding effleurage stroke to cover the rest of your pet's body. For the limbs, begin close to where the limb joins the body and stroke down the limb toward the paw. Stroke each limb several times, so you cover every inch of skin. This light continuous stroke increases circulation and, at the same time, calms your pet.

WARM-UP REMEDY FOR ACTIVE PETS

Just as we have to warm up and loosen our muscles before working out, it's also helpful to improve performance and prevent injury for active pets who spend their days running, hiking with their owners, or simply bouncing off the walls as kittens and puppies seem to do. Your active pet will benefit greatly from a regular warm-up to relax the limbs and increase the circulation to all muscles.

1. Using the heel of your hand, vigorously rub the large muscles, including the neck, shoulders, buttocks, and thighs, in a circular motion (either clockwise or counterclockwise is fine). Spend at least 30 seconds on each area, then move to the next area.

2. Gently lift and knead the muscles all over your pet's body with each hand as if you were kneading bread. Spend extra time on the thigh area, which tends to be tight.

3. Move your hands down to the legs, near where they meet the body, and gently roll each leg between your hands as you move them down toward the paws. This stimulates the blood flow.

4. Finish by rubbing each paw between your fingers and then gently bending and flexing the paws.

STIFF AND SORE JOINT PET MASSAGE REMEDY

For pets with soreness and stiffness caused by exertion, inactivity, or aging, the Stiff and Sore Joint Pet Massage Remedy can help generate more limberness and alleviate pain. Begin with light-to-medium pressure and then progress to deeper compression if your pet is comfortable. If you start massaging too hard, the muscles will tighten up, and your pet will want to get up and move away. Each animal has its own preference for how much pressure to use and where it feels best. So be extra sensitive and try to tune in to your pet's subtle facial and bodily reactions.

1. Place the palms of your hands on or around the joint to warm up the area for about 10 seconds. Then gently apply pressure using both hands (fingertips for smaller animals) all around the joint. Apply compression, count to three, release, and repeat. Compress at least twice in each spot. Try to cover the entire area around the joint. This helps move fluids through the muscle and relieves tension surrounding the joint. Do this for all joints that are sore or stiff.

2. For a stiff back, place the fingertips of both hands on the muscles on either side of the spine at the base of the neck. Apply firm pressure and then make small circles in a clockwise direction for 5 seconds. Move your fingers down about an inch and repeat applying pressure and small circles. Continue this all the way down to the tail. This acupressure technique can release tension in the back and relieve muscle spasms. If you hit an area that makes your pet tense up, it may be a sore spot or possible trigger point. Just lighten your pressure or move your fingers down to another area.

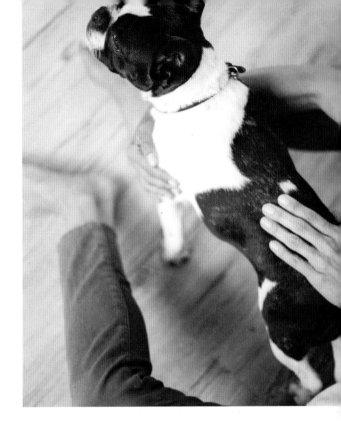

"I LOVE MY PET" EAR REFLEXOLOGY REMEDY

....

Animals have reflexology points in their ears just as we do! By stimulating reflex points in the ears, you can relax and invigorate your pet's entire body. It's easy to do anytime your pet is sitting on your lap or snuggling up close to you.

1. Hold the tops of your pet's ears between your thumb and index finger.

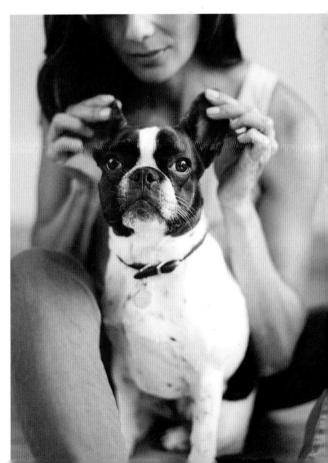

2. Gently massage small circles from the base of the ear down to the lobe. Try not to bend the ear.

3. Hold each ear with your fingers on the outside and your thumb gently inside the ear. Start at the base of your pet's ear, gently pulling outward all the way around until you reach the tip of the ear.

ANTI-ANXIETY ACUPRESSURE
PET REMEDY

Acupressure is just as effective on dogs and cats as it is on us. Animals' bodies also contain numerous acupressure points, some of which, when stimulated, can relieve anxiety and calm aggressive or skittish behavior. These points are places where energy (*chi*) accumulates. By applying pressure to these areas on your pets, you can open congested energy pathways, so your pet is more balanced and relaxed. These points are located in similar places in dogs, cats, and horses. (These are called "purr points" on cats.)

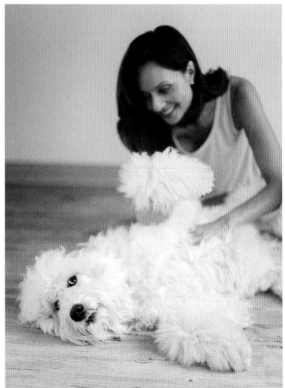

1. *"Highest Spring point" (HT1) point:* This point is located under the armpits. The best way to find this point is to have your pet lie on its back and gently stroke the armpit area with your hand, following the direction of the hair from front to back. When your pet is relaxed, place your fingertips in the deepest spot in the center of the armpit crease, about halfway from the front to back. Apply gentle but firm pressure and hold this point for 10 seconds. Then make small circles in one direction and then the other for 1 minute. Repeat on the other armpit.

2. *"Hundred Meetings" (GV20) point:* This point is located in the central indentation in the middle of the top of the head, exactly halfway between

the ears. Press your fingertips on this point for 10 seconds and then make back-and-forth motions for another 20 seconds. This point calms the spirit and clears the mind.

3. *"Heart's Hollow" (B15) point:* This point is located on either side of the spine, in the small indentations where the top of the fifth rib meets the vertebra. Apply gentle but firm pressure and hold this point for 10 seconds. Then make small circles in one direction and then the other for 1 minute. This supports the heart, calms, and cools.

4. *"Spirit Gate" (H7) point:* This point is located on the outside back of the lower front leg. Bend the wrist and feel for the large, natural depression formed slightly above and behind the wrist crease. Apply firm pressure for 30 seconds and then repeat on the other leg. This point helps heart problems, stabilizes emotions, and calms.

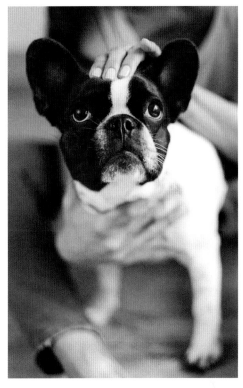

Hundred Meetings Point

DAILY PET MASSAGE REMEDY

A 5-minute routine that is a combination of several pet massage techniques, the Daily Pet Massage Remedy is something you can do every day to increase blood and lymph circulation and relax every part of your pet's body. I recommend doing it at night, before going to bed. Massage is a soothing way to send your pet off to dreamland feeling secure and loved, and it can help *you* tune out the worries of the day and unwind.[12]

1. Place one hand at the base of your pet's neck and the other on its lower back. Hold for 30 seconds.

2. Place your palms flat on your pet's head and make long, slow effleurage strokes all the way down the neck, the length of the spine, and the tail. You can stroke both hands together or alternate hands. Keep your hands on the muscles on either side of the spine, never directly on the spine. Repeat several times, gradually increasing pressure if your pet likes it.

3. Continue the effleurage stroke moving from the spine down the chest. Do this as many times as you need to cover the entire body.

4. Effleurage each of the legs, starting close to where the limb meets the body, moving toward the paws.

5. Rub each paw between your fingers, and then gently bend and flex the paws.

6. Place your index and middle fingers on the muscles on either side of the spine, close to the base of the neck, and apply firm pressure. Make small clockwise circles for 5 seconds, then move an inch down the spine and repeat. Continue all the way down the spine to the tail. This relaxes the entire back.

7. Finally, place the index and middle finger of one hand on the indentation in the middle of the top of the head, exactly halfway between the ears (the "Hundred Meetings," GV20, acupressure point). Press your fingertips on this point for 10 seconds, then make back-and-forth motions for another 20 seconds. This relieves anxiety and relaxes every part of your pet's body.

> *Lots of people talk to animals. . . . Not very many listen,*
> *though. . . . That's the problem.*
>
> —BENJAMIN HOFF, *The Tao of Pooh*

IT IS HEALTH THAT IS
THE REAL WEALTH
AND NOT PIECES OF
GOLD AND SILVER.

—MAHATMA GANDHI

ACKNOWLEDGMENTS

There are many people who helped me bring this book to fruition and to whom I owe my deepest gratitude and appreciation. To begin with, I want to thank each and every one of the massage instructors and clients I had the opportunity to work with over the years. You have all taught me that the power of touch is truly reciprocal and it does transform your life.

Special thanks to my literary agent, Andrew Stuart, for your guidance and support on this project from concept to completion. Thanks to Claudia Boutote at HarperElixir for your excitement, encouragement and support; my insightful editor and #1 cheerleader, Libby Edelson, for your hard work, thoughtful edits, and invaluable help with my manuscript; Nancy Hancock, for taking an early interest in my book; and to everyone at HarperCollins who has touched this book along the way, including Melinda Mullin, Adrian Morgan, Aida Colar, Jennifer Jensen, and Lisa Zuniga.

Thanks to my fantastic photographer, Arna Bajraktarevic, for capturing the essence of this book with her beautiful images. I am grateful to Dr. Mehmet Oz and all the producers at *The Dr. Oz Show* who have given me a platform to bring touch therapy into mainstream media and increase public awareness. Thank you, Natalie Schnaitmann and Linda Klein at City of Hope in Los Angeles, for giving me the opportunity to bring touch therapy to people who need it the most.

I appreciate everyone who shared their insights about touch therapy with me, including Dr. Myles Spar, Dr. Tiffany Field, Dr. Jerrilyn Cambron, Shay Reider, Tim Allen, Hollye Jacobs, Lauren Cates, and Dacher Keltner.

I am beyond grateful for the love and support of my dearest friends and family who kept me sane and without whom I could never have found the clarity or commitment to write. Thank you, Justine Roddick and Tina Schlieske, for offering a sanctuary away from home where I could write in peace. Thank you, Cheryl Nizam, Helen and Richard Kluck, Marilyn and Steven Ebbin, Elizabeth and Paloma Colling, James Vacarro, Taylor Mitchell, Bean, and the staff at Evolation Yoga SB.

Finally, my overwhelming love and deepest gratitude goes to my husband, Luke, who spent countless hours reading every word I wrote and flying solo with our boys for days on end. To Jackson, Cassidy, and Tanner, thank you for being my guinea pigs and models. I love you more than words can ever express.

NOTES

Introduction

1. Peggy Orenstein, "The Way We Live Now: Stress Test," *New York Times Magazine,* June 29, 2008, http://www.nytimes.com/2008/06/29/magazine/29wwlnlede-t.html.

2. Richard Knox, "For Many Americans, Stress Takes a Toll on Health and Family," *NPR .org,* July 7, 2014; http://www.npr.org/sections/health-shots/2014/07/07/323351759/for-many -americans-stress-takes-a-toll-on-health-and-family.

3. "Research," *American Massage Therapy Association,* https://www.amtamassage.org/research/.

4. Kirsten Fawcett, "Massage as Medicine: Massage Therapy Is Increasingly Being Embraced as an Alternative Medical Treatment," *U.S. News & World Report,* February 12, 2015, http://health .usnews.com/health-news/health-wellness/articles/2015/02/12/massage-as-medicine.

5. Rose Adams, Barb White, and Cynthia Beckett, "The Effects of Massage Therapy on Pain Management in the Acute Care Setting," *International Journal of Therapeutic Massage and Bodywork* 3(1) (2010): 4–11.

6. David J. Linden, *Touch: The Science of Hand, Heart, and Mind* (New York: Viking, 2015), 197.

7. Tiffany Field, *Touch* (Cambridge, MA: MIT Press, 2001).

8. Kory Floyd, "What Lack of Affection Can Do to You: We're Facing a Crisis of Skin Hunger, and It Has Real Consequences," *Psychology Today,* August 31, 2013, https://www .psychologytoday.com/blog/affectionado/201308/what-lack-affection-can-do-you.

9. Urban Dictionary, s.v. "skin hunger," http://www.urbandictionary.com/define .php?term=skin+hunger.

Chapter 1: Touch-Therapy Techniques and Tools

1. M. Majchrzycki, P. Kocur, and T. Kotwicki, "Deep-Tissue Massage and Nonsteroidal Anti-Inflammatory Drugs for Low Back Pain: A Prospective Randomized Trial," *Scientific World Journal,* February 23, 2014, doi: 10.1155/2014/287597.

2. S. J. Kim, O. Y. Kwon, and C. H. Yi, "Effects of Manual Lymph Drainage on Cardiac Autonomic Tone in Healthy Subjects," *International Journal of Neuroscience* 119(8) (2009): 1105–17.

3. Carol A. Samuel and Ivor S. Ebenezer, "Exploratory Study on the Efficacy of Reflexology for Pain Threshold and Tolerance Using an Ice-Pain Experiment and Sham TENS Control," *Complementary Therapies in Clinical Practice* 19(2) (May 2013): 57–62.

4. James L. Oschman, *Energy Medicine: The Scientific Basis* (London: Churchill Livingstone, 2000).

5. J. Post-White et al., "Therapeutic Massage and Healing Touch Improve Symptoms in Cancer," *Integrative Cancer Therapy* 2(4) (December 2003): 332–44.

Chapter 2: Touch More, Stress Less: The Stress–Touch Connection

1. M. A. Diego et al., "Aggressive Adolescents Benefit from Massage Therapy," *Adolescence* 37(147) (Fall 2002): 597–607.

2. Bloomberg.com. Visual Data. 2013; http://www.prnewswire.com/news-releases/affluent -in-the-us-australia-and-japan-have-the-highest-stress-in-the-world-brazil-and-hong-kong-the -lowest-73101697.html.

3. Wendy Rogers, *Social Psychology: Experimental and Critical Approaches* (Maidenhead, UK: Open University Press, 2003), 110.

4. Lisa Miller, "Prescription Drug Abuse Is a By-Product of Modern American Life," *Prescription Drug Abuse*, eds. Margaret Haerens and Lynn M. Zott (Detroit: Greenhaven Press, 2013). Opposing Viewpoints. "Listening to Xanax," *New York Magazine* 18 (March 2012). *Opposing Viewpoints in Context.* Web. 9 Sept. 2015; http://ic.galegroup.com/ic/ovic/ViewpointsDetails Page/DocumentToolsPortletWindow?displayGroupName=Viewpoints&action=2&catId=& documentId=GALE%7CEJ3010865218&source=Bookmark&u=jpasj&jsid=3f5027313108 3063196f6d0fd789922a.

5. Benedict Carey, "Evidence That Little Touches Do Mean So Much," *New York Times,* February 22, 2010, http://www.nytimes.com/2010/02/23/health/23mind.html?_r=0.

6. Carey, "Evidence That Little Touches."

7. Tiffany Field et al., "Massage Therapy Reduces Pain in Pregnant Women, Alleviates Prenatal Depression in Both Parents, and Improves Their Relationships," *Journal of Bodywork and Movement Therapy* 12(2) (April 2008): 146–50.

8. Tiffany Field, *Touch* (Cambridge, MA: MIT Press. 2001), 36.

9. Dacher Keltner, *Born to Be Good: The Science of a Meaningful Life* (New York: Norton, 2009), 182.

10. Matt Richtel, "Your Brain on Computers: Attached to Technology and Paying a Price," *New York Times,* June 6, 2010, http://www.nytimes.com/2010/06/07/technology/07brain .html?_r=0.

11. Aaron Saenz, "Are We Too Plugged In? Distracted vs. Enhanced Minds," *SingularityHUB,* August 26, 2010, http://singularityhub.com/2010/08/26/are-we-too-plugged-in-distracted -vs-enhanced-minds/.

12. Mark Hyman, "Five Ways to Never Be Stressed Again," *Dr. Mark Hyman,* July 3, 2013; http://drhyman.com/blog/2013/04/26/five-ways-to-never-be-stressed-again/.

13. Peggy Orenstein, "The Way We Live Now: Stress Test," *New York Times Magazine,* June 29, 2008, http://www.nytimes.com/2008/06/29/magazine/29wwlnlede-t.html.

14. Roberta Lee, *The SuperStress Solution* (New York: Random House, 2010).

15. "Stress in America: Survey 2013," *American Psychological Association,* http://www.apa.org /news/press/releases/stress/2013/highlights.aspx.

16. Lawrence Murphy and Theodore Schoenborn, eds., "Stress Management in Work Settings," *Centers for Disease Control,* NIOSH Publication #87–111, http://www.cdc.gov/niosh /pdfs/87-111.pdf.

17. http://www.dailymail.co.uk/health/article-2250106/Stress-bad-heart-smoking-cigarettes -day.html#ixzz2FWKaSYsN.

18. U.S. Department of Health and Human Services, Centers for Disease Control and Prevention. "Summary Health Statistics for US Adults: National Health Interview Survey, 2012." Series 10, No. 260. http://www.cdc.gov/nchs/data/series/sr_10/sr10_260.pdf

19. R. Loeppke et al., "Health and Productivity as a Business Strategy: A Multiemployer Study," *Journal of Occupational and Environmental Medicine* 51(4) (April 2009): 411–28.

20. Wharton School of Business, "Stressed Out By Work? You're Not Alone," *Knowledge@ Wharton,* October 30, 2014, http://knowledge.wharton.upenn.edu/article/stressed-work-youre -alone/.

21. Linda Beck, "Anxiety Can Bring Out the Best: Researchers Prescribe Just Enough Stress to Ace Life's Tests; Too Little Is Lazy," *Wall Street Journal,* June 18, 2012, http://www.wsj.com /articles/SB10001424052702303836404577474451463041994.

22. "Stress," *University of Maryland Medical Center,* http://umm.edu/health/medical/reports /articles/stress.

23. E. Epel et al., "Stress May Add Bite to Appetite in Women: A Laboratory Study of Stress-Induced Cortisol and Eating Behavior," *Psychoneuroendocrinology* 26(1) (January 2001): 37–49.

24. Ruth Werner, "'Jangled' Adults: Touch and the Stress Response System," *Massage and Bodywork Magazine,* February/March 2006, http://www.massagetherapy.com/articles/index.php/article_id/1162/Jangled-Adults.

25. "Stress in America: Survey 2013," *American Psychological Association,* http://www.apa.org/news/press/releases/stress/2013/highlights.aspx.

26. Mina Westman, "Crossover of Stress and Strain in the Family and Workplace," in Pamela L. Perrewe and Daniel C. Ganster, eds., *Historical and Current Perspectives on Stress and Health,* vol. 2, Research in Occupational Stress and Well-being (Bingley, UK: Emerald, 2002), 143—81.

27. V. Engert et al., "Cortisol Increase in Empathic Stress Is Modulated by Social Closeness and Observation Modality," *Psychoneuroendocrinology* 45 (July 2014): 192–201.

28. Jeffrey R. Edwards and Nancy P. Rothbard, "Mechanisms Linking Work and Family: Clarifying the Relationship Between Work and Family Constructs," *Academy of Management Review* 25(1) (January 2000): 178–99.

29. Engert et al, "Cortisol Increase in Empathic Stress."

30. Michael Price, "Alone in the Crowd: Sherry Turkle Says Social Networking Is Eroding Our Ability to Live Comfortably Offline," *American Psychological Association* 42(6) (June 2011): 26, http://www.apa.org/monitor/2011/06/social-networking.aspx.

31. Carolyn Gregoire, "How Our Sense of Touch Affects Everything We Do," *Huffington Post,* January 20, 2015, http://www.huffingtonpost.com/2015/01/20/neuroscience-touch_n_6489050.html.

32. Field, *Touch,* 1.

33. Nora Brunner, "The Power of Touch: In a High-Tech World It Pays to Reach Out," *Body Sense,* Autumn/Winter, 2009, http://www.massagetherapy.com/articles/index.php/article_id/1666/The-Power-of-Touch.

34. Brunner, "The Power of Touch."

35. Diana Spechler, "The Power of Touch: How Physical Contact Can Improve Your Health," *Huffington Post,* May 14, 2013, http://www.huffingtonpost.com/2013/05/14/the-power-of-touch-physical-contact-health_n_3253987.html.

36. Rogers, *Social Psychology,* 110.

37. George H. Colt, "The Magic of Touch: Massage's Healing Powers Make It Serious Medicine," *Life,* August 1997.

38. S. M. Jourard and J. E. Rubin, "Self-Disclosure and Touching: A Study of Two Modes of Interpersonal Encounter and Their Inter-Relation," *Journal of Humanistic Psychology* 8(1) (Spring 1968): 39–48.

39. James W. Prescott, "The Origins of Human Love and Violence," *Pre- and Perinatal Psychology Journal* 10(3) (Spring 1996): 143–88.

40. Brunner, "The Power of Touch."

41. Gregoire, "How Our Sense of Touch."

42. Mic Hunter and Jim Struve, *The Ethical Use of Touch in Psychotherapy* (Thousand Oaks, CA: Sage, 1998).

43. Field, *Touch,* 2–3.

44. Ofer Zur and Nola Nordmarken, "To Touch or Not to Touch: Exploring the Myth of Prohibition on Touch in Psychotherapy and Counseling," *Zur Institute,* 2011, http://www.zurinstitute.com/touchintherapy.html.

45. Ashley Montagu, *Touching: The Human Significance of the Skin,* 3rd ed. (New York: Harper & Row, 1986).

46. Field, *Touch,* 57.

47. David J. Linden, *Touch: The Science of Hand, Heart, and Mind* (New York: Viking, 2015), 5.

48. Keltner, *Born to Be Good,* 180, 194.

49. Matthew Hertenstein et al., "Touch Communicates Distinct Emotions," *Emotion* 6(3) (August 2006): 528–33.

50. Spechler, "The Power of Touch."

51. Edmund T. Rolls, "The Orbitofrontal Cortex and Reward," *Cerebral Cortex* 10(3) (2000): 284–94.

52. Keltner, *Born to Be Good,* 182.

53. Keltner, *Born to Be Good,* 187.

54. Alberto Gallace and Charles Spence, "The Science of Interpersonal Touch: An Overview," *Neuroscience and Biobehavioral Reviews* 34(2) (February 2010): 246–59.

55. Linden, *Touch,* 153–54.

56. Tiffany Field, "Massage Therapy Effects," *American Psychologist* 53(12) (December 1998): 1270–81.

57. Keltner, *Born to Be Good,* 197–98.

58. Hertenstein, "Touch Communicates Distinct Emotions."

59. Keltner, *Born to Be Good,* 197.

60. Gregoire, "How Our Sense of Touch Affects Everything We Do," *Huffington Post,* January 20, 2015.

61. Field, *Touch,* 67–70.

62. Tiffany Field, Miguel Diego, and Maria Hernandez-Reif, "Preterm Infant Massage Therapy Research: A Review," *Infant Behavior and Development* 33(2) (April 2010): 115–24.

63. Tiffany Field et al., "Autistic Children's Attentiveness and Responsivity Improve After Touch Therapy," *Journal of Autism and Developmental Disorders* 27(3) (June 1997): 333–38.

64. National Institutes of Health, National Center for Complementary and Integrative Health, "Massage Therapy," January 27, 2015, http://www.massagetherapy.com/learnmore/benefits.php.

65. If you're interested in learning more about the studies for each problem, I highly suggest you visit the Touch Research Institute website (http://www6.miami.edu/touch-research/) for the most recent information.

66. Suzanne C. Segerstrom and Gregory E. Miller, "Psychological Stress and the Human Immune System: A Meta-Analytic Study of 30 Years of Inquiry," *Psychological Bulletin* 130(4) (July 2004): 601—30.

Chapter 3: Hands on You: DIY Self-Care for Every Body

1. Leon Kreitzman, *The 24-Hour Society* (London: Profile, 1999).

2. Nancy O'Brien, "5 Dimensions of Self-Caring That Heal Healthcare: The Foundation of an Experience Management Strategy." *Experience in Motion,* 2010, http://experienceinmotion.net/wp-content/uploads/2011/05/Executive-Summary-5-Dimensions-of-Self-Caring.pdf.

3. O'Brien, "5 Dimensions of Self-Caring."

4. Linda Carroll, "American Anxiety: Why We're Such a Nervous Nation," *Today.com,* August 20, 2012, http://www.today.com/health/american-anxiety-why-were-such-nervous-nation-953854.

5. Laura Schocker, "This Is Your Body On Stress," *Huffington Post,* April 5, 2013.

6. S. J. Kim, O. Y. Kwon, and C. H. Yi, "Effects of Manual Lymph Drainage on Cardiac Autonomic Tone in Healthy Subjects," *International Journal of Neuroscience* 119(8) (2009):1105–17.

7. Andrew Weil, "Aromatherapy," *DrWeil.com,* http://www.drweil.com/drw/u/ART03205/Aromatherapy.html.

8. Salynn Boyle, "100 Million Americans Have Chronic Pain: New Study Shows That Pain Costs Billions of Dollars a Year in U.S."; WebMD Health News: http://www.webmd.com/pain-management/news/20110629/100-million-americans-have-chronic-pain.

9. D. C. Cherkin et al., "A Comparison of the Effects of 2 Types of Massage and Usual Care on Chronic Low-Back Pain: A Randomized, Controlled Trial," *Annals of Internal Medicine* 155(1) (2011): 1–9.

10. Maria Hernandez-Reif et al., "Lower Back Pain Is Reduced and Range of Motion Increased After Massage Therapy," *International Journal of Neuroscience* 106(3–4) (2001): 131–45.

11. M. Majchrzycki, P. Kocur, and T. Kotwicki, "Deep-Tissue Massage and Nonsteroidal Anti-Inflammatory Drugs for Low Back Pain: A Prospective Randomized Trial," *Scientific World Journal* (February 23, 2014): Article ID 287597.

12. Maryam Eghbali et al., "The Effects of Reflexology on Chronic Low Back Pain Intensity in Nurses Employed in Hospitals Affiliated with Isfahan University of Medical Sciences," *Iranian Journal of Nursing and Midwifery Research* 17(3) (March–April 2012): 239–43.

13. Christian Nordqvist, "Fatigue: Why Am I So Tired?" *Medical News Today,* June 17, 2015, http://www.medicalnewstoday.com/articles/248002.php.

14. "Chronic Fatigue: In-Depth Report," *New York Times,* http://www.nytimes.com/health /guides/disease/chronic-fatigue-syndrome/print.html.

15. American Academy of Pain Medicine. "AAPM Facts and Figures on Pain." http://www .painmed.org/patientcenter/facts_on_pain.aspx.

16. Christopher Quinn, Clint Chandler, and Albert Moraska, "Massage Therapy and Frequency of Chronic Tension Headaches," *American Journal of Public Health* 92(10) (October 2002): 1657–61.

17. H. Hemmingway and M. Marmot, "Psychological Factors in the Aetiology and Prognosis of Coronary Heart Disease: Systematic Revision of Prospective Cohort Studies," *British Medical Journal* 318(7196) (1999): 1460–67.

18. "Heart Disease and Stress: What's the Link?" *Web*MD, October 8, 2014, http://www .webmd.com/heart-disease/guide/stress-heart-disease-risk.

19. U.S. Dept. of Health & Human Services, National Heart, Lung, and Blood Institute. "Your Guide to a Healthy Heart," http://www.nhlbi.nih.gov/health/resources/heart/healthy -heart-guide-html.

20. Zahra Zare, Hooman Shahsavari, and Mahin Moeini, "Effects of Therapeutic Touch on the Vital Signs of Patients Before Coronary Artery Bypass Graft Surgery," *Iranian Journal of Nursing and Midwifery Research* 15(1) (Winter 2010): 37–42 (PMCID: PMC3093033).

21. F. S. Dhabhar et al., "Stress-Induced Redistribution of Immune Cells—From Barracks to Boulevards to Battlefields: A Tale of Three Hormones—Curt Richter Award Winner," *Psychoneuroendocrinology* 37(9) (September 2012): 1345–68.

22. Saul A. McLeod, "Stress, Illness and the Immune System," *SimplyPsychology,* 2010, http:// www.simplypsychology.org/stress-immune.html.

23. Heena Patel, "Insomnia Plagues More Women Than Men," *Society for Women's Health Research,* June 24, 2014, http://swhr.org/resource/insomnia-plagues-more-women-than-men/.

24. Kristyn Kusek Lewis, "Massage: It's Real Medicine," *CNN.com,* March 8, 2007, http:// www.cnn.com/2007/HEALTH/03/08/healthmag.massage/.

25. M. L. Chen et al., "The Effectiveness of Acupressure in Improving the Quality of Sleep of Institutionalized Residents," *Journals of Gerontology Series A: Biological Sciences and Medical Sciences* 54 (8) (August 1999): M389–94.

26. Bryan Raudenbush, "WJU Professor and Students Find Jasmine Odor Leads to More Restful Sleep, Decreased Anxiety and Greater Mental Performance," Wheeling Jesuit University, http://www.wju.edu/about/adm_news_story.asp?iNewsID=539.

27. Melanie Greenberg, "Why We Gain Weight When We're Stressed—And How Not To: The Psychology and Biology of Stress-Related Overeating and Weight Gain," *Psychology Today,* August 28, 2013, https://www.psychologytoday.com/blog/the-mindful-self-express/201308/why -we-gain-weight-when-we-re-stressed-and-how-not.

Chapter 4: Women's Remedies: Nurture the Nurturers

1. "Anxiety: In-Depth Report," *New York Times,* http://www.nytimes.com/health/guides /symptoms/stress-and-anxiety/print.html.

2. Joan Borysenko, *Fried: Why You Burn Out and How to Revive* (Carlsbad, CA: Hay House, 2011).

3. Tiffany Field et al., "Pregnant Women Benefit from Massage Therapy," *Journal of Psychosomatic Obstetrics and Gynaecology* 20(1) (March 1999): 31–38; "Massage Therapy Effects on Depressed Pregnant Women," *Journal of Psychosomatic Obstetrics and Gynaecology* 25(2) (June 2004): 115–22.

4. Field et al., "Pregnant Women Benefit from Massage Therapy."

5. Tiffany Field et al., "Massage Therapy Reduces Pain in Pregnant Women, Alleviates Prenatal Depression in Both Parents and Improves Their Relationships," *Journal of Bodywork and Movement Therapy* 12(2) (April 2008): 146–50.

6. Sylvia Cataldo Oportus et al., "Clinical Study: Lymph Drainage in Pregnant Women," *Nursing Research and Practice* 2013 (October 22, 2013): Article ID 364582.

7. Fatemeh Dabiri and Arefeh Shahi, "The Effect of LI4 Acupressure on Labor Pain Intensity and Duration of Labor: A Randomized Controlled Trial," *Oman Medical Journal* 29(6) (November 2014): 425–29, PMID: 25584160.

8. Michele Borba, "7 Tricks to Help Stressed Moms Chill Out," *Today.com,* January 26, 2012, http://www.today.com/parents/7-tricks-help-stressed-moms-chill-out-1C7397996.

9. "Parenting: Being Supermom Stressing You Out?" *American Psychological Association,* May 2011, http://www.apa.org/helpcenter/supermom.aspx.

10. Borba, "7 Tricks."

11. Richard E. Harris et al., "Traditional Chinese Acupuncture and Placebo (Sham) Acupuncture Are Differentiated by Their Effects on Opioid Receptors (MORs)," *Neuroimage* 47 (3) (September 2009): 1077–85.

12. National Sleep Foundation (online). "White Paper: Consequences of Drowsy Driving." http://sleepfoundation.org/white-paper-consequences-drowsy-driving.

13. International Journal of Clinical Acupuncture. http://www.intmedsolutions.com/facial -rejuvenation-acupuncture-for-anti-aging/.

14. U.S. Census Bureau, *Population Survey: Female Population by Age, Sex, Race and Hispanic Origin,* March 2002.

15. Kristyn Kusek Lewis, "Massage: It's Real Medicine," *CNN.com,* March 8, 2007, http:// www.cnn.com/2007/HEALTH/03/08/healthmag.massage/.

16. Barbara and Kevin Kunz, "Reflexology and Menopause," *Reflexology Research Project Presents,* http://www.reflexology-research.com/.

17. T. Oleson and W. Flocco, "Randomized Controlled Study of Premenstrual Symptoms Treated with Ear, Hand, and Foot Reflexology," *Obstetrics and Gynecology* 82(6) (December 1993): 906–11.

18. H. Y. Chiu et al., "Effects of Acupuncture on Menopause-Related Symptoms and Quality of Life in Women in Natural Menopause: A Meta-Analysis of Randomized Controlled Trials," *Menopause Journal* 22(2) (February 2015): 234–44.

19. Shelley Emling, "Menopause Symptoms: Is 'The Change' Destroying Your Memory?" *HuffingtonPost.com,* last updated January 23, 2014, http://www.huffingtonpost.com/2013/01/03 /menopause-symptoms-memory-loss_n_2397936.html.

Chapter 5: Men's Remedies: Massage Away Your Problems

1. Mark Greene, "The Lack of Gentle Platonic Touch in Men's Lives Is a Killer," *The Good Men Project,* November, 4, 2013, http://goodmenproject.com/featured-content/megasahd-the-lack -of-gentle-platonic-touch-in-mens-lives-is-a-killer/.

2. Bridget Murray-Law, "Why Do Men Die Earlier?" *American Psychology Association* 42(6) (June 2011), http://www.apa.org/monitor/2011/06/men-die.aspx.

3. Janelle Davis, "New Survey Finds Majority of Men Avoid Preventive Health Measures," *AAFP,* June 19, 2007, http://www.aafp.org/media-center/releases-statements/all/kits/20070619 .html.

4. Interview with Myles D. Spar, M.D., M.P.H., Director of Integrative Medicine at Venice Family Clinic's Simms/Mann Health and Wellness Center, January 11, 2015.

5. Dacher Keltner, *Born to Be Good: The Science of a Meaningful Life* (New York: Norton, 2009), 182.

6. Greene, "The Lack of Gentle Platonic Touch."

7. Spar, interview.

8. Spar, interview.

9. Murray-Law, "Why Do Men Die Earlier?"

10. Sung-Hak Cho, Soo-Han Kim, and Du-Jin Park, "The Comparison of the Immediate Effects of Application of the Suboccipital Muscle Inhibition and Self-Myofascial Release Techniques in the Suboccipital Region on Short Hamstring," *Journal of Physical Therapy Science* 27(1) (January 2015): 195–97.

11. "Prostate Cancer In-Depth Report." New York Times (online). http://www.nytimes .com/health/guides/disease/prostate-cancer/print.html.

12. "Reflexology and the Prostate," *Bauneholm School of Reflexology* (Denmark), https:// pacificreflexology.com/abstract/Men.

13. K. Nunes, H. Labazi, and C. Webb, "New Insights into Hypertension-Associated Erectile Dysfunction." Current Opinion in Nephrology and Hypertension. March 2012-Volume 21-Issue 2-p 163–170. (U.S. National Library of Medicine—National Institutes of Health).

14. http://www.webmd.com/erectile-dysfunction/guide/erectile-dysfunction-basics.

15. Sun Jianhua, "The Comparison of Curative Effects Between Foot Reflexology and Chinese Traditional Medicine in Treating 37 Cases with Male's Sexual Dysfunction," China Reflexology Symposium Report (Beijing: China Reflexology Association, 1996), 75–77.

Chapter 6: Hands on Your Partner: Enhance Intimacy with Touch

1. Elizabeth and Charles Schmitz, "Why Touch Is So Important in a Loving Marriage," *Huffington Post,* November 16, 2013, http://www.huffingtonpost.com/2013/11/16/sex-how -important-is-it_n_4275969.html.

2. A. K. Gulledge, M. H. Gulledge, and R. F. Stahmannn, "Romantic Physical Affection Types and Relationship Satisfaction," *American Journal of Family Therapy* 31(4) (2003): 233–42.

3. Brené Brown, *Daring Greatly: How the Courage to Be Vulnerable Transforms the Way We Live, Love, Parent, and Lead* (New York: Gotham, 2012).

4. Gulledge, Gulledge, and Stahmannn, "Romantic Physical Affection Types."

5. Wendy Rogers, *Social Psychology: Experimental and Critical Approaches* (Maidenhead, UK: Open University Press, 2003), 110.

6. Melissa Duclos, " 'I Get Touched a Lot': Why I Decided to Pay for Cuddling," *Salon.com,* January 17, 2015, http://www.salon.com/2015/01/18/i_get_touched_a_lot_why_i_decided_to _pay_for_cuddling/.

7. Luciana Gravotta, "Be Mine Forever: Oxytocin May Help Build Long-Lasting Love," *Scientific American,* February 12, 2013, http://www.scientificamerican.com/article/be-mine -forever-oxytocin/.

8. "Touching Helps Couples Reduce Stress," *Reuters Health,* January 9, 2009, http://www .reuters.com/article/2009/01/09/us-touching-stress-idUSTRE5085A120090109.

9. "Marriage Linked to Better Survival in Middle Age: Study Highlights Importance

of Social Ties During Midlife," *Springer Select,* January 10, 2013, http://www.springer.com /about+springer/media/springer+select?SGWID=0-11001-6-1401342-0.

10. A. Gallace and C. Spence, "The Science of Interpersonal Touch: An Overview," *Neuroscience and Biobehavioral Reviews* 34(2) (February 2010): 246–59.

11. Petra Boynton, "Goodnight Kiss Is a 'Thing of The Past,'" *Telegraph,* October 14, 2012, http://www.telegraph.co.uk/women/mother-tongue/9607602/Goodnight-kiss-is-a-thing-of -the-past.html.

12. Carolyn Castiglia, "Non-Sexual Physical Affection Is the Key to a Happy Marriage," *Babble.com,* 2014, http://www.babble.com/relationships/non-sexual-physical-affection-is-the -key-to-a-happy-marriage/.

13. Gravotta, "Be Mine Forever."

14. Andrea Horn, "Touch as an Interpersonal Emotion Regulation Process in Couples' Daily Lives: The Mediating Role of Psychological Intimacy," *Personality and Social Psychology Bulletin* 39(10) (October 2013): 1373–85.

15. "Female Sexual Dysfunction," *Web*MD, http://www.webmd.com/women/guide/sexual -dysfunction-women.

16. "Acupressure," *Susan G. Komen,* http://ww5.komen.org/BreastCancer/Acupressure.html.

17. Paul Engelhardt et al., "Acupuncture in the Treatment of Psychogenic Erectile Dysfunc- tion: First Results of a Prospective Randomized Placebo-Controlled Study," *International Journal of Impotence Research* 15(5) (October 2003): 343–46.

18. M. H. Rapaport, P. Schettler, and C. Breese, "A Preliminary Study of the Effects of a Single Session of Swedish Massage on Hypothalamic-Pituitary-Adrenal and Immune Function in Normal Individuals," *Journal of Alternative Complementary Medicine* 16(10) (October 2010): 1079–88.

19. Norine Dworkin-McDaniel, "Touching Makes You Healthier," *CNN.com,* January 5, 2011, http://www.cnn.com/2011/HEALTH/01/05/touching.makes.you.healthier.health/.

20. W. Collinge, J. Kahn, and R. Soltysik, "Promoting Reintegration of National Guard Veterans and Their Partners Using a Self-Directed Program of Integrative Therapies: A Pilot Study," *Military Medicine* 177(12) (December 2012): 1477–85.

21. U. Chatchwan et al., "Effects of Thai Traditional Massage on Pressure Pain Threshold and Headache Intensity in Patients with Chronic Tension-Type and Migraine Headaches," *Journal of Alternative and Complementary Medicine* 20(6) (June 2014): 486–92.

22. V. Buttagat et al., "Therapeutic Effects of Traditional Thai Massage on Pain, Muscle Tension and Anxiety in Patients with Scapulocostal Syndrome: A Randomized Single-Blinded Pilot Study," *Journal of Bodywork and Movement Therapies* 16(1) (January 2012): 57–63.

23. Natthakarn Chiranthanut, Nutthiya Hanprasertpong, and Supanimit Teekachunhatean, "Thai Massage and Thai Herbal Compress Versus Oral Ibuprofen in Symptomatic Treatment of Osteoarthritis of the Knee: A Randomized Controlled Trial," *BioMed Research International* (September 1, 2014): Article ID 490512.

Chapter 7: Calm Kids: Touch Remedies for Kids of All Ages

1. Ashley Montagu, *Touching: The Human Significance of the Skin,* 3rd ed. (New York: Harper & Row, 1986).

2. Tiffany Field, "Massage Therapy Facilitates Weight Gain in Preterm Infants," *Current Directions in Psychological Science* 10(2) (April 2010): 51–54.

3. Sharon Heller, *The Vital Touch: How Intimate Contact with Your Baby Leads to Happier, Healthier Development* (New York: Holt, 1997).

4. Alvin Powell, "Children Need Touch and Attention, Harvard Researchers Say," *Harvard University Gazette,* April 9, 1998, http://news.harvard.edu/gazette/1998/04.09/ChildrenNeedTou .html.

5. Shirley Vanderbilt, "Children and Massage: A Powerful Combination," *Body Sense Magazine,* Spring 2003, http://www.massagetherapy.com/articles/index.php/article_id/470/Children-and-Massage.

6. J. A. Spencer et al., "White Noise and Sleep Induction," *Archives of Disease in Children* 65(1) (1990): 135–37.

7. Tiffany Field, Miguel Diego, and Maria Hernandez-Reif, "Preterm Infant Massage Therapy Research: A Review," *Infant Behavior Development* 33(2) (2010): 115–24.

8. T. Field, S. Schanberg, and F. Scafidi et al., (1986), "Tactile/Kinesthetic Stimulation Effects on Preterm Neonates," *Pediatrics,* Vol. 77, 654–58; http://www6.miami.edu/touch-research/InfantMassage.html.

9. Infant Massage USA: International Association of Infant Massage; http://www.infantmassageusa.org/learn-to-massage-your-baby/benefits-of-infant-massage/.

10. T. Field, M. Diego, and M. Hernandez-Reif et al., "Moderate Versus Light Pressure Massage Therapy Leads to Greater Weight Gain in Preterm Infants." *Infant Behavior and Development.* Dec. 2006; Vol. 29(4): 574–78. Published online 2006 Nov 13. doi: 10.1016/j.infbeh.2006.07.011

11. Field, "Massage Therapy Facilitates Weight Gain."

12. B. Çetinkaya and Z. Basbakkal, "The Effectiveness of Aromatherapy Massage Using Lavender Oil as a Treatment for Infantile Colic," *International Journal of Nursing Practice* 18(2) (April 2012): 164–69.

13. "Caring for Your Baby and Young Child: Birth to Age 5," 6th Edition (Copyright © 2015 American Academy of Pediatrics). https://healthychildren.org/English/ages-stages/baby/crying-colic/Pages/Colic.aspx.

14. Çetinkaya and Basbakkal, "The Effectiveness of Aromatherapy Massage Using Lavender Oil."

15. Maryanne Hanley, "Therapeutic Touch with Preterm Infants: Composing a Treatment," *Explore (New York)* 4(4) (July–August 2008): 249–58.

16. Shay Beider, "Touching the Future: Gentle Massage for Children," *Massage Magazine,* November 2006, 63.

17. Tiffany Field et al., "Massage Reduces Anxiety in Child and Adolescent Psychiatric Patients," *Journal of the American Academy of Child and Adolescent Psychiatry* 31(1) (January 1992): 125–31.

18. A. Escalona et al., "Brief Report: Improvements in the Behavior of Children with Autism Following Massage Therapy," *Journal of Autism and Developmental Disorders* 31(5) (October 2001): 513–16.

19. Tiffany Field et al., "Children with Asthma Have Improved Pulmonary Function After Massage Therapy," *Journal of Pediatrics* 132(5) (May 1998): 854–58.

20. T. Field, O. Quintino, M. Hernandez-Reif, and G. Koslovsky, (1998), "Adolescents with Attention Deficit Hyperactivity Disorder Benefit from Massage Therapy," *Adolescence* 33, 103–108. S. Khilnani, T. Field, M. Hernandez-Reif, and S. Schanberg, (2003). "Massage Therapy Improves Mood and Behavior of Students with Attention-Deficit/Hyperactivity Disorder," *Adolescence* 38, 623–38.

21. Maria Hernandez-Reif et al., "Cerebral Palsy Symptoms in Children Decreased Following Massage Therapy," *Early Child Development and Care* 175(5) (2005): 445–56.

22. Maria Hernandez-Reif et al., "Children with Down Syndrome Improved in Motor Function and Muscle Tone Following Massage Therapy," *Early Child Development and Care* 176(3–4) (May 2006): 395–410.

23. Tina Allen, *A Modern-Day Guide to Massage for Children* (Blue Miso Books, 2014).

24. Beider, "Touching the Future."

25. Mimi Ko Cruz, "No Hugs? Get a Grip, Kids Say," *Los Angeles Times,* February 12, 1998, http://articles.latimes.com/1998/feb/12/local/me-18438.

26. "Tennessee Legislature Approves Bill Banning 'Gateway Sexual Activity,'" Sexuality Information and Education Council of the United States, April, 2012, http://www.siecus.org/index.cfm?fuseaction=Feature.showFeature&featureID=2170.

27. American College Health Association, *National College Health Assessment, Spring 2013 Reference Group Executive Summary.*

Chapter 8: Caring for the Elderly: A Labor of Love

1. Kimberly Palmer, "The Cost of Caring for Aging Parents," *U.S. News & World Report,* August 27, 2014, http://money.usnews.com/money/personal-finance/articles/2014/08/27/the-cost-of-caring-for-aging-parents.

2. Leeann Doherty, "The Stresses of Caring for an Elderly Parent," *New Hampshire Magazine,* June 2014, http://www.nhmagazine.com/June-2014/The-Stresses-of-Caring-for-a-Parent/.

3. Carolyn Gregoire, "How Our Sense of Touch Affects Everything We Do," *Huffington Post,* January 20, 2015, http://www.huffingtonpost.com/2015/01/20/neuroscience-touch_n_6489050.html.

4. Gregoire, "How Our Sense of Touch Affects Everything We Do."

5. A. Abdulla et al., "Evidence-Based Clinical Practice Guidelines on Management of Pain in Older People," *Age and Ageing* 42(2) (2013): 151–53.

6. A. I. Perlman et al., "Massage Therapy for Osteoarthritis of the Knee: A Randomized Controlled Trial," *Archives of Internal Medicine* 166(22) (December 11–25, 2006): 2533–38.

7. "Research Shows Massage Therapy Lowers Stress and Aggression in Dementia," *Massage Magazine,* December 10, 2010, http://www.massagemag.com/research-shows-massage-therapy-lowers-stress-and-aggression-in-dementia-patients-8375/.

8. J. Kutner, M. Smith, and L. Corbin, *Massage Therapy vs. Simple Touch to Improve Pain and Mood in Patients with Advanced Cancer: A Randomized Trial.* Published in final edited form as: *Ann Intern Med* 149(6), September 16, 2007: 369–79.

9. Alexia Elejalde-Ruiz, "Thriving Through Touch: Gentle Massage Helps Older People with Low Mobility Improve in Body and Mind," *Chicago Tribune,* December 14, 2011, http://articles.chicagotribune.com/2011-12-14/health/sc-health-1214-senior-health-massage-20111214_1_touch-research-institute-massage-therapists-tiffany-field.

10. Tiffany Field et al., "Elder Retired Volunteers Benefit from Giving Massage Therapy to Infants," *Journal of Applied Gerontology* 17(2) (June 1998): 229–39.

11. "Research Roundup: Ageing and Massage," *American Massage Therapy Association,* October 2014, https://www.amtamassage.org/research/Massage-Therapy-Research-Roundup/Research-Roundup.html.

12. "Ageism in America: As Boomers Age, Bias Against the Elderly Becomes Hot Topic," *NBC News,* September 7, 2004, http://www.nbcnews.com/id/5868712/ns/health-aging/t/ageism-america/#.

13. "Consumer Survey Fact Sheet," *American Massage Therapy Association,* October 2014, https://www.amtamassage.org/research/Consumer-Survey-Fact-Sheets.html?src=navdropdown.

14. "Ageism in America."

15. Eric Nagourney, "Why Am I So Cold?" *New York Times,* November 15, 2012, http://www.nytimes.com/2012/11/15/booming/why-do-i-feel-colder-as-i-get-older.html?_r=0.

16.   E. M. DiNucci, "Energy Healing: A Complementary Treatment for Orthopaedic and Other Conditions," *Orthopaedic Nursing* 24(4) (July–August 2005): 259–69.

17.   University of Maryland Medical Center, "Therapeutic Touch," http://umm.edu/health/medical/altmed/treatment/therapeutic-touch#ixzz3RBzZXTbB.

Chapter 9: Healing Remedies: Touch During Illness

1.   "Consumer Survey Fact Sheet," *American Massage Therapy Association,* October 2014, https://www.amtamassage.org/research/Consumer-Survey-Fact-Sheets.html?src=navdropdown.

2.   S. T. Keir and J. R. Saling, "Pilot Study of the Impact of Massage Therapy on Sources and Levels of Distress in Brain Tumor Patients," *BMJ Supportive and Palliative Care* 2(4) (2012): 363–66.

3.   M. Toth et al., "Massage Therapy for Patients with Metastatic Cancer: A Pilot Randomized Controlled Trial," *Journal of Alternative and Complementary Medicine* 19(7) (July 2013): 650–56; Meghan J. Thomason and Christopher A. Moyer, "Massage Therapy for Lyme Disease Symptoms: A Prospective Case Study," *International Journal of Therapy Massage Bodywork* 5(4) (2012): 9–14.

4.   A. M. Castro-Sánchez et al., "Benefits of Massage-Myofascial Release Therapy on Pain, Anxiety, Quality of Sleep, Depression, and Quality of Life in Patients with Fibromyalgia," *Evidence-Based Complementary Alternative Medicine* (2011): 561753.

5.   J. A. Coan, H. S. Schaefer, and R. J. Davidson, "Lending a Hand: Social Regulation of the Neural Response to Threat," *Psychological Science* 17(12) (December 2006): 1032–39.

6.   "Arthritis," *National Center for Chronic Disease Prevention and Health Promotion,* http://www.cdc.gov/chronicdisease/resources/publications/aag/arthritis.htm.

7.   Tiffany Field et al., "Rheumatoid Arthritis in Upper Limbs Benefits from Moderate Pressure Massage Therapy," *Complementary Therapy Clinical Practice* 19(2) (May 2013): 101–3.

8.   Tiffany Field et al., "Neck Arthritis Pain Is Reduced and Range of Motion Is Increased by Massage Therapy," *Complementary Therapy Clinical Practice* 20(4) (November 2014): 219–23.

9.   "Massage," American Cancer Center, http://www.cancer.org/acs/groups/cid/documents/webcontent/acspc-041660-pdf.pdf; B. Cassileth and A. J. Vickers, "Massage Therapy for Symptom Control: Outcome Study at a Major Cancer Center," *Journal of Pain Symptom Management* 28(3) (September 2004): 244–49; Karagozoglu S., Kahve E. "Effects of Back Massage on Chemotherapy-Related Fatigue and Anxiety: Supportive Care and Therapeutic Touch in Cancer Nursing," *Appl Nurs Res* 2013 Nov; 26(4): 210-17. doi: 10.1016/j.apnr.2013.07.002. Epub 2013 Sep 20. PubMed PMID: 24055114.

10.   Kristyn Kusek Lewis, "Massage: It's Real Medicine" *CNN.com,* March 8, 2007, http://www.cnn.com/2007/HEALTH/03/08/healthmag.massage/.

11.   Diana Khoury, "NIH Research Grant Funds Study on the Effects of Reflexology and Cancer," March 22, 2013, http://www.washingtonreflexology.org/2013/03/nih-research-grant-funds-study-on-the-effects-of-reflexology-cancer/.

12.   Maria Hernandez-Reif et al., "Breast Cancer Patients Have Improved Immune Functions Following Massage Therapy," *Journal of Psychosomatic Research* 57(1) (July 2004): 45–52.

13.   Hollye Jacobs, *The Silver Lining: A Supportive and Insightful Guide to Breast Cancer* (New York: Atria, 2014). Interview.

14.   "Therapeutic Massage and Diabetes," American Massage Therapy Association, December 21, 2002, https://www.amtamassage.org/articles/3/MTJ/detail/1774.

15.   D. F. Elson and M. Meredith, "Therapy for Type 2 Diabetes Mellitus," *Wisconsin Medical Journal* 97(3) (March 1998): 49–54.

16.   Tiffany Field, "Massage Therapy for Infants and Children," *Journal of Developmental and Behavioral Pediatrics* 16(2) (April 1995): 105–11.

17.   Tiffany Field et al., "Massage Therapy Lowers Blood Glucose Levels in Children with Diabetes Mellitus," *Diabetes Spectrum* 10 (1997): 237–39.

18. "Opportunities and Challenges in Digestive Diseases Research: Recommendations of the National Commission on Digestive Diseases." U.S. Department of Health and Human Services National Institutes of Health, NIH Publication No. 08-6514 March 2009. http://www.niddk.nih.gov/about-niddk/strategic-plans-reports/Documents/NCDD%20Research%20Plan/NCDD_04272009_ResearchPlan_CompleteResearchPlan.pdf.

19. "Therapeutic Massage," Johns Hopkins Medicine, Integrative Medicine and Digestive Center, http://www.hopkinsmedicine.org/integrative_medicine_digestive_center/services/therapeutic_massage.html.

20. A. R. Mitchinson et al., "Acute Postoperative Pain Management Using Massage as an Adjuvant Therapy: A Randomized Trial," *Archives of Surgery* 142(12) (December 2007): 1158–67; discussion 1167.

21. "Questions and Answers About Fibromyalgia," National Institute of Arthritis and Musculoskeletal and Skin Diseases, July 2014, http://www.niams.nih.gov/Health_Info/Fibromyalgia/default.asp.

22. Castro-Sánchez et al., "Benefits of Massage-Myofascial Release Therapy."

Chapter 10: Kneaded Pets: Pets Need Touch Too

1. "Seizure Alert/Response Dogs," Service Dog Central, www.servicedogcentral.org/content/node/491.

2. Carolyn M. Willis et al., "Olfactory Detection of Human Bladder Cancer by Dogs: Proof of Principle Study," *British Medical Journal* 329(7468) (September 25, 2004): 712.

3. Michael W. Fox, *The Healing Touch for Dogs: The Proven Massage Program* (New York: Newmarket, 2004), 2–3.

4. Marty Becker, *The Healing Power of Pets: Harnessing the Amazing Ability of Pets to Make and Keep People Happy and Healthy* (New York: Hyperion, 2002).

5. Glen Levine, "Pet Ownership and Cardiovascular Risk: A Scientific Statement From the American Heart Association." American Heart Association, *Circulation*. Published online May 9, 2013. http://circ.ahajournals.org/content/early/2013/05/09/CIR.0b013e31829201e1.full.pdf+html

6. Amanda B. Coakley and Ellen K. Mahoney, "Creating a Therapeutic and Healing Environment with a Pet Therapy Program," *Complementary Therapy Clinical Practice* 15(3) (August 2009): 141–46.

7. Fox, "The Healing Touch for Dogs," pp. 12–16. "All About Animal Massage," 2013. http://allaboutanimalmassage.com. Hourdebaigt, Jean-Pierre, LMT. "Canine Massage: A Complete Reference Guide." Dogwise Publishing, 2004.

8. Norine Dworkin-McDaniel, "Touching Makes You Healthier," *CNN.com,* January 5, 2011, http://www.cnn.com/2011/HEALTH/01/05/touching.makes.you.healthier.health/.

9. James A. Serpell, "Animal Companions and Human Well-Being: An Historical Exploration of the Value of Human-Animal Relationships," in Aubrey H. Fine, ed., *Handbook on Animal-Assisted Therapy: Theoretical Foundations and Guidelines for Practice* (San Diego: Academic, 2000), chap. 1.

10. Tracy McVeigh, "Not Just Horsing Around . . . Psychologists Put Their Faith in Equine Therapies," *Guardian,* February 25, 2012, http://www.theguardian.com/society/2012/feb/26/horses-therapists-stress-autism-addiction.

11. McVeigh, "Not Just Horsing Around."

12. For more information on animal therapies, visit the International Alliance of Animal Therapists and Healers (IAATH), http://www.iaath.com.

REFERENCES

Field, Tiffany. *Complementary and Alternative Therapies Research*. Washington, DC: American Psychological Association, 2009.

————. *Touch*. Cambridge, MA: MIT Press, 2001.

Fox, Michael W. *The Healing Touch for Dogs: The Proven Massage Program*. New York: Newmarket, 2004.

Hess, Samantha. *Touch: The Power of Human Connection*. 2nd ed. Fulcrum Solutions LLC, 2014.

Hourdebaigt, Jean-Pierre. *Canine Massage: A Complete Reference Manual*. Wenatchee, WA: Dogwise, 2004.

Jacobs, Hollye. *The Silver Lining: A Supportive and Insightful Guide to Breast Cancer*. New York: Atria, 2014.

Keltner, Dacher. *Born To Be Good: The Science of a Meaningful Life*. New York: Norton, 2009.

Klaus, Marshall H., John H. Kennell, and Phyllis H. Klaus. *Bonding: Building the Foundations of Secure Attachment and Independence*. Boston: Addison-Wesley, 1995.

Linden, David J. *Touch: The Science of Hand, Heart, and Mind*. New York: Viking, 2015.

Liu, Zhanwen, and Liang Liu, eds. *Essentials of Chinese Medicine*. London: Springer, 2010.

McClellan, Stephanie, and Beth Hamilton. *The Ultimate Stress-Relief Plan for Women*. New York: Free Press, 2010.

Montagu, Ashley. *Touching: The Human Significance of the Skin*. 3rd ed. New York: Harper & Row, 1986.

Schneider McClure, Vimala. *Infant Massage: A Handbook for Loving Parents*. 3rd rev. ed. New York: Bantam, 2000.

Spar, Myles D., and George E. Munoz. *Integrative Men's Health*. New York: Oxford University Press, 2014.

INDEX

54; Swedish, 20, 22, 72, 92, 101, 105–6, 131, 138–40, 171, 189–91; Thai partner massage, 8, 22, 131, 140–43. *See also* touch-therapy techniques

meditation, 5, 60

memory remedy, 111–13

men: health remedies for, 119–25; nonsexual touch to enhance relationships, 127–43; touch isolation and health issues of, 115–18

menopause and PMS management remedies, 106–13

metabolism, 78

"Middle of a Person" point, 99

mindfulness, 5

moms' health and remedies, 95–101

Mood Swings Reflexology Remedy, 107–8

myofascial release, 23, 119, 208–9

nausea remedies, 86–87

NBA "touch-bonded" teams, 32–33

neck reflex area, 89, 108

neck reflex point, 69

neuropeptide S, 39

neurotransmitters (stress hormones), 39

New Walkers Massage Remedy, 172–73

night-sweat remedy, 109–11

"No Holding Hands Bill" (Tennessee, 2012), 175–76

nonsexual touch: cuddling, 128–29; enhancing relationship remedies, 131–43; importance to a healthy relationship, 127–31; male "touch isolation" lack of, 116–17

occipital ridge, 68

orbitofrontal cortex (OFC), 40, 47

oxytocin ("feel-good") hormone, 5

Partners 5-Minute Reflexology Remedy, 131, 136–38

Partners Back and Shoulder Deep-Tissue Remedy, 131, 133–36

Partners Full-Body Swedish Massage Remedy, 131, 138–40

Partners Intimacy Acupressure Remedy, 131–32

Partners Thai Massage Remedy, 140–43

"Peaceful Sleep" point, 100

pets: anti-anxiety acupressure, 224–25; massage for, 219–23, 225–26; reflexology for, 223–

24; tension and stress absorbed by, 215–16; touch benefits for you and your, 216–19

pineals reflex area, 79

pregnancy remedies: anti-nausea, 86–87; back-pain, 91–92; headache, 89–90; health benefits of the, 83, 85; massage, 19; pregnancy precautions for, 85; stress-relief, 92, 94; swollen feet and ankles, 88–89

prostate or urinary problem remedy, 121–22

prostate reflex area, 121–22

PTSD (posttraumatic stress disorder), 36, 49

reflexology: anti-anxiety, 56, 57, 183; anti-fatigue, 66; anti-headache, 69–71, 89–91; anti-nausea, 87; back-pain, 62–63, 91; cancer patients, 205–6; Cold Feet (Poor Circulation) Remedy, 191–93; 5-Minute Interlocking Hand Reflexology Remedy, 176–77; heart problems, 72; immunity-boosting, 183; Intimacy Acupressure Remedy use of, 132; Mood Swings Reflexology Remedy, 107–8; overview of, 19–20, 21; Partners 5-Minute Reflexology Remedy, 131, 136–38; for pets, 223–24; prostate or urinary problem, 121–22; Relaxing Incentive Reflexology Remedy, 178–79; stress-relief, 94; studies on the benefits of, 1; weight issues, 79. *See also* touch-therapy techniques

Reflexology Sox, 8

relaxation response, 39–40

Relaxing Incentive Reflexology Remedy, 178–79

reproductive organs reflex area, 107–8

Romanian orphanage report (1990), 17–18

"Rushing Door" (SP12) points, 132

school "touch avoidance" policies, 44, 175–76

"Sea of Energy" (CV6) point, 78, 79, 124

"Sea of Tranquility" point, 56, 65

"Sea of Vitality" (B23 and B47) points, 123

self-care (DIY, do-it-yourself), 8, 53–54, 118

Self-Myofascial Release (SMR), 23, 119

side-to-side ankle loosening, 137

"Si Shien Chong" point, 98

"skin hunger." *See* touch hungry ("skin hunger")

sleep remedies, 76–77, 99–101

solar plexus reflex point, 57, 58, 66